# Lost

# Lost

*Sharing my life with Brain Injury*

## Karen Betts

authorHOUSE®

*AuthorHouse*™
*1663 Liberty Drive*
*Bloomington, IN 47403*
*www.authorhouse.com*
*Phone: 1-800-839-8640*

*First published by AuthorHouse    09/21/2011*

*ISBN: 978-1-4567-8583-3 (sc)*

*Printed in the United States of America*

*Any people depicted in stock imagery provided by Thinkstock are models, and such images are being used for illustrative purposes only.*
*Certain stock imagery © Thinkstock.*

*This book is printed on acid-free paper.*

For Aaron,

Who lost part of his life, this is to help him understand what happened and the implications his brain injury has had.

To anyone who has suffered a brain injury and for those who cared for them.

# Content

# Prologue

We all go along in life living day to day in this rat race, complacent and predictable in how we get. Not really looking at great length at what is important until it is taken away from us without our control.

The things we take for granted especially those we live with and are close to. I never thought I could feel such pain, until the day I lost my dad to cancer in March 2008. In the past I've lost grandparents, felt sad at their passing. But when it's your parents it's something completely different. Somewhere in the subconscious of your mind you think they are going to live forever, nothing can prepare you for what you experience when they go. Although as a family we knew dad was dying while he was still alive there was part of me that kept thinking he'll be ok. Waiting in the hospital relative's room on that day was the longest I have known. Mum and I sat reminiscing whilst Aaron (my husband) my brother and sister in law sat with dad, waiting for him to go. I just couldn't bring myself to be in the same room whilst he took his last breath, if I stayed away part of it felt it wasn't happening. Suddenly hearing Aaron shout for the ward sister I knew he'd gone. Looking up at the clock it had just struck five. From that moment on life would never be the same and I never wanted to step foot in a hospital again.

Since dad's death part of me has gone as well, I got threw it mainly because of Aaron. Dad was always there now he's not getting use to that I've found has been the hardest. Whenever the phone rings at home I half expect him to be on the other end calling for a chat when he'd had one too many whiskies. Aaron has been my rock since dad died he's the one that has kept me going, made me laugh when I got down. Seeing the memories and smiling along with the keepsake box I treasure but then feeling sad as it's now the only contact left with him. Not sure if it's the recent events that have made me miss him more. You never get used to them not being there but you adapt to the situation, keep going the best way you can, giving support to other loved ones. There's a saying "what does not kill you makes you stronger" and believe me no truer word has been spoken.

On 28th April 2009 my life changed again without warning after Aaron collapsed at home early one morning. Later finding out he suffered a brain injury (sub-arachnoid haemorrhage) our lives will now never be the same. Thank goodness he's still alive, but the battles we have both faced have tested us to the limits. I am still waiting for the day I get my husband back, if I ever will.

This story is based on the events relating to Aaron's brain injury and the journey of recovery he has made. But it mainly focuses on the journey I have gone through, in the dual role of wife and carer. From day one I have kept diaries mainly to help Aaron when he is able to understand what has happened. They have also helped me therapeutically overcome some dark days. All the trials and tribulations, the mental, emotional and physical traumas I've had to deal with. The up's and downs feeling like you are travelling through a dark tunnel and at one point not seeing the light at the end. The denial, shock and panic thinking "please god let him live" to the relief and elation on "he's going to be ok" hoping that he will continue to make progress, to the realisation of "him not getting back to his old self".

Then comes acceptance knowing your lives will be completely different from now on. The hardest feeling I've had to deal with was guilt, not blaming myself for what happened but I tended to make things harder for myself. Trying to do everything and not ask for help. Feeling guilty because this tragedy happened to Aaron and maybe there could have been more to prevent it. I read somewhere that you feel neither "married nor single", a feeling of being trapped with nowhere to run, torn of what to do, stay and deal with the situation the best way you can or give up. It's like going through the grieving process but without the death, something that I could not begin to explain. Wondering and hating myself for thinking would it have been better all round if Aaron hadn't of made it. At least the grieving process would have had some form of meaning. I feel as if I have gone through every marriage vow in the last 2 years. In sickness and in health, for better for worse and very nearly till death us do part. Going from wife to carer giving it my all, feeling completely lost.

I knew nothing about brain injury like most of us until this happened to Aaron. Still learning every day though as new challenges arise. Over the last two years brain injury has been my life, day in day out just about every waking breath. You'd think I'd be an expert by now, far from it. Constantly trying to gain more knowledge, educate myself so that I can alert others to this horrific injury that affects so many people.

Research indicates that approximately over 8,000 people in the UK each year are affected by sub-arachnoid haemorrhage. 75% of these turn out to be brain aneurysms the majority of these cases will often occur without warning. Sufferers can make a good recovery but some may suffer neurological or physical disabilities. This is why it is important for us to be aware of this type of injury.

Not to sound too daunting it is estimated that between 10-15% of people will die before they can get to a hospital and up to 50% can still die within a month of a haemorrhage. This is the reality of it.

Because there is little or no warning that a bleed to the brain will occur most people will not know what the problems is, individuals may have symptoms of a severe headache, vomiting, sensitivity to light and becoming confused, some may even collapse. Those that attend hospital without collapsing in the first instance still may not know and sometimes hospital diagnosis is often missed. It is not appreciated that the warning signs prior to a brain haemorrhage occur in about 50% of individuals. Knowing this makes it a scary thought.

There are two types of brain injury firstly Traumatic Brain Injury (TBI). This is when the head can receive a severe blow caused by an accident or assault. The effects of this are wide and depend on a number of factors such as the severity and location of the injury. It can also cause a host of physical, cognitive and emotional effects and the outcome can range from complete recovery to permanent disability or even death. The second is Acquired Brain Injury (ABI) this is any injury that has occurred by events after birth, derived from a stroke, haemorrhage or infection. Like TBI it usually affects cognitive, physical, emotional, social and independent functions. Anyone with a brain injury may have difficulty controlling, coordinating and communicating their thoughts and actions, but they still retain their intellectual abilities. They may however find it difficult to express themselves in a manner intelligible to others, which can make the sufferer of a brain injury more vulnerable.

Brain injury can be especially difficult for family and friends mainly understanding what has happened and as time goes on the sufferer may go on to look fine physically, but cognitively could take at lot longer. Often family and friends find it hard to know what to say to the sufferer, not sure if to ask if they are ok? Or behave as though nothing has changed. However anyone who has suffered a brain injury may find it difficult to express themselves, talk about what problems they are facing, this may lead to them becoming depressed and isolated. Mood swings such as anger, frustration and irritability can be difficult for family and friends to cope with, but the sufferer might not be aware that their behaviour has changed.

So before I go onto to share with you the last couple of years I think it's only fair to tell you a little about me and Aaron, who was 39 at the time of his brain injury. Reading on you'll discover we were just ordinary people living ordinary lives, as time went on, then seeing the difference it has made not just on his life but my life as well.

The first time I met Aaron was at a friend's wedding in July 2003. I knew the bride as we started work together in 2000 for the same police force. Aaron and the groom had known each since they were at school. The last thing I was looking for on the day of the wedding was another relationship, to tell you the truth I was off men for good at that point. We were somehow thrown together but as time went by we got chatting and he seemed a decent bloke. Couple of months later things were going ok so on Christmas day 2003 we got engaged, quick you may think. After that time flew and before I knew it we had bought a house in Rushden and moved in by March 2004. The only people I knew there at that time were Michelle and Andrew, the couple whose wedding we met at. Plans had been set for getting married on 25th September 2004 at the Guildhall Northampton, never felt so nervous in my life a huge step and hopefully the right one. The day went well Aaron took control to make sure I enjoyed it. All in all looking back one of the memories I treasure is that my dad got to see it.

Aaron himself, well he's a considerate, intelligent and hardworking man and he enjoyed his job. There was a little bit of a perfectionist about Aaron when it came to his work. He has a good circle of friends, two especially Andrew (Ted) and Matthew (Woody) he's always willing to help anyone out. Very independent knows what he wants. He also has his sceptical side but can on occasions be optimistic. On the other hand he can be stubborn, cantankerous, confrontational and opinionated which some thought boarded on him being sarcastic. But at the end of the day life was ok we were making the best of what we had plus he made me laugh. Since his injury Aaron's personality has stayed intact, which is a blessing but he gets more frustrated and agitated with himself and others, his patience has been reduced he becomes more confrontational, especially when challenged. Even though he claims he was like this before his injury his emotions and moods have magnified which can make him at times unpredictable.

Aaron worked as a Health and Safety Advisor when I first met him in 2004 he got a new position in the August with a reputable company, he was there for 5 years until he was made redundant in January 2009. It was a worry Aaron being out of work the mortgage and bills still needed paying, I was the only one working but it wasn't long before Aaron was soon on the lookout for another job. It was the beginning of February 2009 when he went for an interview, being successful he started his new job as a Health and Safety Advisor with a new company on 30th March 2009. As I dropped him off at the train station on his first day I pulled away in the car thinking things were starting to look up again.

The weekend before Aaron's injury he went away for the weekend to Birmingham with the lads to see The Specials in concert, he was so excited he'd arranged everything from the tickets, hotel and transport. It was not until after his injury that I discovered from his friends that he was acting strange over the weekend they noted that he was the only one being sick, dropping things and not being able to focus when picking them up, becoming sensitive to light. No one really made an issue of it for who was to know what was going to happen. The general consensus was that he's had too much to drink or had eaten something that had not agreed with him. They can remember driving home on the Sunday afternoon noticing that Aaron was driving towards the white lines in the middle of the road. Getting home safely, blissfully unaware of what the weekend held. Once at home Aaron went straight to bed with a headache I just thought it was the after effects of the weekend, lack of sleep, too much alcohol not knowing any difference. He got up after a couple of hours claiming he still felt rough so took it easy for the rest of the night. I must admit I was a bit peeved with him, part of me felt he deserved feeling bad.

27th April 2009 I had taken the day off as it was my dad's birthday. Just wanted a little time off for me maybe go shopping, didn't need an excuse to do that. The week before I attended an interview at work, which for me was promotion. Hearing I got the job in a way this was my treat, no harm in that as long as I don't go too mad on the Radley's. Aaron went to work as usual but by lunch time he was home still complaining of a headache. Not thinking anything was wrong he took some tablets lay on the sofa trying to sleep it off. I left him to it, carried on making the most of my day off before work the next morning. By mid afternoon a supermarket run was called for, Aaron decided to come with me he seemed fine claiming the headache had gone off a bit. So with bags in hand we carried on as normal. We were out for about an hour, got back, unpacked and settled for the evening. Nothing much occurred that night, cooked dinner, watched a bit of TV nothing out of the ordinary on a week night. Preparations were made for the morning lunches were packed as we both knew it was an early start. As I prepared for bed after showering I can still remember the last thing I said to Aaron that night before we fell asleep it was "how's your head" he replied "still niggling" no I love you, not imagining for one moment that the next day I would live to regret not saying it.

# Chapter One

*His life in their hands*

————◄❧►————

2 8th April 2009—I lay in bed listening to the morning alarm play to itself thinking, I should get up but trying to get my body to move from under the warm duvet was another matter. Why is it you feel more tired when you know you have to work, but when you are off you are wide awake? I should have got up an hour earlier to go into work to do some overtime, but the thought of that did not appeal so I stayed in bed. I looked over at the clock, It was 0515am, feeling like the middle of the night still. Eventually Aaron turned the alarm off got up, threw on his dressing gown and went downstairs to put the kettle on. No words had been exchanged between us at this point, but that was nothing unusual as it takes me a while to come round in a morning. Still trying to find the motivation to move, but kept thinking just another couple of minutes.

On his way back upstairs Aaron went into the bathroom turned on the shower to get it warmed up before jumping in. I was still laying there five minutes had passed when I heard a loud noise come from the bathroom. The only way to describe the sound was like someone throwing plastic bottles in the bath very loudly. Shouting to Aaron to ask if all was ok, no reply I shouted again still no reply by now feeling really hot, I jumped out of bed ran into the bathroom as instinct told me something wasn't right. On opening the door I found Aaron lying in the bath, shower curtain pulled from the rail his head near the taps, making this dreadful noise that I can't describe but it's a noise that will haunt me forever. The shower was still running, steam was building up and I just froze for a split second. As he lay there unconscious I could hear myself screaming at him to wake up but all I could hear was my heart pounding through my chest getting louder and louder. It was then the noise stopped, panic set in. Running to get the phone to call for an ambulance still not sure what had happened. The operator took some details and asked to describe what happened. "I don't know" "he's not breathing" found myself rambling at this stage. The operator was my only life line at that point. He then asked if I could get Aaron out of the bath, no chance he was soaking wet and I wasn't even sure if he was dead or alive or what damage had been done. There was no way I could even attempt to lift him out. The operator advised me to go and knock up a neighbour to help as Aaron needed to be taken out of the bath ready for the paramedics, who were on their way. Not knowing many people in the street didn't help also the majority of them were elderly, there was only one person I could think of. Running out of the house bare footed leaving the front door wide open I frantically knocked on the house next door but one where Tanya lived. The seconds felt endless, lights then went on, door opened. Words came out and I tried to explain what had happened, without hesitation Tanya followed me. Straight away she took control trying to keep me calm, telling me to get dressed whilst she went to see Aaron. Being a former nurse she knew what to do. As Tanya felt for a pulse she looked up and said there was one, "thank god" I thought he was still alive. All he needs to do now was hang on.

Seconds later the paramedics arrived they immediately began to work on Aaron, the house was manic. I was in the bedroom getting dressed so I was ready to go with Aaron. I was shaking from head to toe, feeling physically sick imagining what the hell was going on. I heard a car pull up outside, looking out of the window seeing Aaron's parents arrive after I called them earlier.

Coming out of the bedroom Aaron had been put into a chair and was being carried downstairs he looked dreadful, so pale oxygen mask on his face they quickly escorted him to the waiting ambulance. I didn't even get time to ask how he was or what had happened. It didn't even cross my mind that this could have been related to the last few days and the headaches Aaron had suffered.

With ambulance doors securely shut I had to follow behind with his parents as there was no room in the back for me due to there being an extra paramedic that had arrived shortly after. I began to feel even more afraid not being able to go with him. The nearest hospital was Kettering about a thirty minute drive. A feeling of nausea sweep over me as soon as I got into the car I opened the window and took deep breaths. We had been travelling for about ten minutes when in the distance I could see the ambulance pull over in a lay by. My immediate reaction was "he's dead" that's why they've stopped? My hand was on the door handle ready to jump out of the car and run over to see what happened but by the time we found somewhere to park the ambulance was back on route. Not knowing if he was dead or alive the remainder of the journey to the hospital seemed never ending. I must admit I have never felt as scared as I did then. I refused to believe he could be dead and that I may now be facing my life as a widow.

We drove into the hospital grounds getting dropped off just outside A&E, at reception we were told to go straight to the relative's room, someone will be along shortly. The room wasn't all that big, it was so hot in there I could hardly breathe it felt really claustrophobic. By now there was about six of us in there. It felt like I was looking at myself from the other side of the room that this wasn't really happening it was all a nightmare and I will soon wake up. A sense of silence fell in the room I think it was just pure shock. The doctor came in along with a nurse and handed me Aaron's wedding ring and dressing gown, saying that they had to put Aaron to sleep as when he came round he was becoming agitated. They were not sure at this point exactly what was going on, all they knew was there seemed to be something going on in his head. A CT scan needed to be done to ascertain just what the problem was. Something you never want to hear the words seemed to echo through my soul, hitting me like a lead weight. What does this mean? Questions were racing through my mind. Not believing that this was actually occurring, a sense of denial on my part.

The doctor went on to say that Aaron suffered a seizure on the way to Kettering, that's why the ambulance stopped. Going on to mentioned the Glasgow Coma Scale (GCS), made no sense to me but in fact this is to ascertain someone's condition. The GCS is scored between 3-15, three being the worse and 15 the best. There are three parameters that determine someone's condition, best eye response, verbal and motor responses. Coma scale of 13 and above correlates to a mild brain injury, 9-12 Moderate and 8—less is severe. Aaron's started as a 15 then reduced to 6. I remember the doctor turning to me and saying "it doesn't look good" feeing suffocated I had to get out of that room. The fresh air hit me like a brick wall unable to come to terms with the realisation of what was happening. What did he mean "it doesn't look good" Aaron wouldn't leave me? Not like this? A few hours ago everything was ok and now? How can things change so quickly? It made no sense. Putting on what rational head I had left knowing I had some phone calls praying this would take my mind off the horror that waits. Staring at my phone not knowing where to start, who do I call first? Work was the main priority for Aaron as well as me. Luckily I had a contact for Aaron's new job they needed to know what was happening. Trying to explain the events of the morning was hard to believe, all I could do was update them when we knew what was going on. Called my brother, with mum not being in the country and dad gone, he was my only family. I needed him here, as soon as he heard what had happened he said he was on his way. Sue my sister in law was seven months pregnant at the time so with the news of Aaron she was coming to the right place if anything happened. Mum was away in the states on holiday. This was the first real break she'd had had since dad died so until I knew what we were dealing with my brother and I decided not to call her.

Trying to compose myself to face whatever was thrown at me I went back inside for any news. The results of the CT scan were in and it revealed that Aaron had had a bleed to the brain. What did this mean? Is it something that can be fixed? Why was there no warning? Being Diagnosed as a Sub-arachnoid Haemorrhage (SAH). This is where blood leaks out of a blood vessel over the surface of the brain, a medical emergency and requires immediate treatment to prevent serious complications and in some cases death. Three quarters of SAH are caused when an aneurysm ruptures. This is a bulge in a blood vessel that is caused by a weakness in the blood vessel wall. Some people are born with aneurysm and never know it, some may not even rupture. But the risk heightens if you smoke, drink excess alcohol and suffer from high blood pressure. 70% of SAH are caused by aneurysms. Once it has burst the aneurysm will often seal itself and bleeding will stop. But the risk of that is if no treatment is sought it may bleed again and this time with serious consequences. With a SAH the blood damages the brain tissue, reduction of blood supply can often cause further brain damage and again in some cases death.

The scan results were being faxed over to the John Radcliffe Hospital in Oxford to see if they could help as Aaron needed specialist treatment. The words became muffled couldn't take in what was being said but I didn't want to miss anything either. Cannot believe that less than 24hrs ago we were both alive and talking now Aaron was fighting for his life. Could not bear thinking about what could happen. Needed to get out for some air as emotions just took over, the tears flowed at that point there was nothing I could do to stop them. What seemed like forever (but was only 20 minutes) we were called back in, Kettering had got a reply from Oxford, with everything crossed we waited for the answer. They had looked at the scans and agreed to take Aaron. A sigh of relief all round suddenly I could see a slight glimmer of hope. We were asked if we would like to see Aaron before he was transported to Oxford as time was now of the essence. Part of me did want to see him but part of me didn't as I wasn't sure what to expect. Walking into the A&E department with my brother and Aaron's family, I saw him lying there with tubes and machines everywhere bleeping. It just did not seem real my legs went I was completely drained. Standing there with a feeling like the whole room was moving at a fast pace and I was the only one standing completely still. Grabbing my brother's arm for support knowing without it I'd fall, looking over at him I saw the tears in his eyes. Praying for Aaron to open his eyes or squeeze my hand, anything to let me know he was still there. The last thing on my mind was the thought of having to say goodbye to him if things took a turn for the worse but by then that was not an option for me, I refused to believe he could die.

I remember one of the nurses came up to me touched my arm and said "it's good news about Oxford, it appears they will only take you if they can help" I knew there and then we had a tough battle on our hands. Filled with determination not to give up I leant down and whispered to Aaron to do the same. A fight was ahead so I put on my outer shield ready for the battle to commence.

Transport was going to take a while so it was now a waiting game. Aaron for the time being had been transferred to the intensive care unit (ICU) until he could be moved. The longer however he was at Kettering the more at risk he was of another bleed occurring. I looked at the clock every five minutes at one point the hand didn't seem to move for half an hour. Suddenly it was action stations, nurses rushing all over the place, getting equipment ready for the journey it was time. I leant over kissed him gently on the cheek and whispered to him to hang on and I would see him soon. It felt like my heart had been ripped apart. What If this was the last time I see him alive? Mad with myself for thinking such a thought I hurried out of the hospital to go home and pack a bag ready to go to Oxford. At home I quickly packed a few things arranged for the animals to be fed and prepared myself for a very long night but trying not to think that far ahead, as the situation could change in a minute. In the forefront of my mind the main concern was hoping he makes the journey.

Good job I wasn't driving to Oxford that afternoon could not have told you much about it my mind was going over and over the last few hours. By mid afternoon we finally arrived at the John Radcliffe Hospital. As we entered the car park we were greeted by a magnificent building. Its stature presented a presence of hope which by now was all I had. Signposted well, we eventually found the NICU (Neuro Intensive Care Unit) at reception we were told that Aaron had just arrived and they were getting him settled. He made it? All he had to do now was hang on a bit longer. Trying to stay positive was really hard as the next few hours were critical.

One of the consultants arrived to take us through to the unit nothing had prepared me for what I saw as we entered the ward. It was nothing I had ever seen before, large open plan, very bright with floor to ceiling windows, equipment that looked like the deck of a space ship. Banks of machines either side of the bed. But it was the staff that I found, especially over the weeks to come that were a credit to their profession the dedication and commitment shown was second to none. It was then I saw Aaron lying there so still, ventilator pumping breath into his lungs. Drips and wires everywhere, laying there his face pale like porcelain, with no bruising or marks anywhere. So hard to identify just how damaged he was. Not a flicker of life, I knew somewhere he was in there, buried but not dead, we were now facing the waiting game. The whole place reminded me of my dad, making a vow to myself not to step foot in a hospital again. It was still so raw wasn't sure at that point who I was grieving for the most. Reality hit me with a sledgehammer within seconds a doctor approached and asked for a word, being escorted into a side room he explained about the bleed to Aaron's head and the damages it could entail. I tried to take in all he was saying but as soon as he spoke I forgot everything. They said they wanted to carry out another scan just to see what they were dealing with. Some people who have suffered brain injury are never the same person they were, that on a number of occasions has been pointed out to me, even to this day. They no longer recognise loved ones simply abandon their family, even their own personality changes forever. That was a possibility with Aaron that we might have to face. Was I ready to deal with that right now? No.

Evening was starting to fall feeling completely drained, couldn't even remember if I'd eaten or drunk anything. Switching on my phone to an array of messages and voice mails knowing this would keep me occupied later.

The hospital was kind enough to provide a room that night, but knowing I wasn't going to get much sleep, if any. All this felt like a nightmare that I was stuck in, not being able to wake up. As I sat by Aaron's side staff told me I needed to take time out and get some rest, easier said than done. If there was any change in Aaron's condition they would come and get me. I lay on the bed wide awake the day kept playing around in my mind. Was there anything different I could have done? It felt like I was going mad. Aaron was fighting for his life in the other room and I had to get some sleep, feeling so helpless sleep was the last thing on my mind.

That night seemed to go on forever, seconds felt like minutes, minutes like hours daylight was nowhere to be found. Sitting in the relative's room trying to read a magazine, watching TV nothing could pacify me. Dawn broke as I watched the sun rise hoping it would bring better news. There had been no change to Aaron's condition over night, which in one sense was good. He's still holding on? Pulling myself together I took a shower and changed my clothes trying to wash of any reminder of the day before. Mid morning came and one of the consultants explained what they were dealing with after they had taken a look at the recent scan. He went on to say Aaron had suffered an Aneurysm. Going on to say they can rupture at any time, causing serious bleeding and damage the brain. To prevent a further bleed they would need to operate by sealing, clamping or coiling the aneurysm. There was also a build up of fluid so a drain was placed in the right hand side of his head to get rid of the excess fluid, seeing that was enough to turn your stomach. It's surprising what you overcome when faced with it.

Afternoon approached, the surgeon came to explain what was to happen next and the risks involved. Aaron had also contracted Pneumonia which made the risk of surgery even higher, but without it there was a risk another bleed could occur. I am so glad that they knew what to do. Whatever the risk was something had to be done or he would die as simple as. So that afternoon they were all set to operate. What was there left for me to do, wander the corridors with the world on my shoulders. No I was to go home, shower, change, eat and just wait for the phone call with good or bad news. By the time he went down it was about half past three. Keeping everything crossed for the next few hours, not being able to think straight imagining all could change again. I started to think of the things I never said to Aaron when I had the chance. So many regrets which is a huge weight to carry.

At home I was not left alone, everyone sculling around keeping me occupied when all I wanted to do was hide and feel sorry for myself. The phone rang it was after six, I froze, my heart must have skipped a beat not being able to pick it up. My friend answered, the look on her face said it all he was out of surgery and all went well considering. It felt as though a huge weight had been lifted, trying not to get too excited as this was only the beginning. They had coiled the aneurysm which would prevent any further bleed. Wasn't sure then whether to laugh or cry, so I did both. One hurdle down no doubt many more to go.

Coiling is a method that has been used since the 1900's and is still the preferred method today without the use of a Craniotomy (incision in the scalp) Coiling is a process of approaching the aneurysm from inside the blood vessel, small metal coils, usually platinum which are inserted through the arteries from the groin to the brain. Once they are in place they are not removed. They prevent blood flow to the aneurysm thus reducing the risk of a re-bleed.

Travelling back to Oxford that day I was filled with elation for the first time, ready for the fight. I could not bear to leave his side for the rest of the day, he was not out of the woods yet there was still a chance that his brain could go into spasms but the medication he was on should prevent this. Being by his side part of me thought he will know I'm there but I was beginning to ache all over, sleep was needed and I had to give in at some point for my own health.

It must have been about ten o'clock when we left the hospital. Arrangements had been made to spend the night at a B&B not far from the hospital. Lying on the bed I have never felt so alone, what I wouldn't give for Aaron to walk through that door then we could get in the car and just go home. Another uncomfortable night still ached from the day before. The thought of going down for breakfast did not appeal to me the thought of food made me feel sick. Took my time getting showered, dressed and packed. There was no one else about that morning everywhere seemed so quiet. Having the dining room to ourselves gave me more time to reflect. No phone calls during the night at least but I was anxious to get to the hospital.

Once there we discovered they had stopped the sedation and were trying to wake Aaron up. So soon I thought? Having mixed feelings as not sure what to expect, what if he woke up and did not recognise me? What if he could not wake up? What ifs were racing through my mind? No one knew at this stage knew if any damage had been caused. So for the rest of the day we waited, talked to him trying to get him to open his eyes. Holding his hand asking him to squeeze it, but nothing the longer this went on the more frightened I became.

As the day went on there was no change, he didn't wake up, squeeze my hand or open his eyes so Aaron was put back to sleep. The pneumonia was causing problems and his oxygen levels were getting low. Terrified for both Aaron and me I saw this as a backward move the only thing to do through the night was to monitor him. Being told not to worry didn't help but reassurance that this sometimes happens. A feeling of being inadequate that day not being any help but no amount of rushing was going the make the situation any better. I had to be patient and let nature take its course. As evening fell again there was nothing more to do so for the first time that night I went home alone.

# Chapter Two

## Feeling lost

————◆◆◆————

April 30th2009—Walking into an empty house where even the silence was deafening made me realise just what the last two days had bought. For a minute standing motionless in the hallway not sure what to do first, which to some may sound meaningless. The silence was interrupted by the cats (Bonnie & Clyde) pounding down the stairs they seemed pleased to see me. I felt guilty not being there the last couple of days but all they wanted was food and a fuss. Once fed the next thing on my agenda was having a long hot shower smelling the hospital on me made me feel sick, standing for ages under the cascade of water frozen like a statute in the bath where only a couple of days ago Aaron was lying there barely alive was hard. Looking around you would not believe what had gone on, especially with the mess that was left behind once the paramedics had been there. Wrapping myself up in my oversized dressing gown feeling a sense of loss, the last time I felt anything like this was when dad died. It was strange Aaron not being there, you'd thought I'd get use to it being as though he was away most nights with work, the difference was I knew this time he would not be coming home tomorrow or the next day. Standing at the lounge door I couldn't even bring myself to sit in there, looking over at the place where Aaron sat night after night knowing that there was a possibility he'd never sit there again. Shutting it away meant I could not accept at the moment what was going on.

Couple of hours passed I was itching to call the hospital to see how Aaron was. On speaking to his nurse for the evening he was settled, no change good in a way. With the dread of another long night ahead my thoughts turned of things to occupy myself. I walked around the house in a daze feeling like a stranger in my own home not having the inclination to do anything. The cats seemed to sense something wasn't right as Bonnie would not leave my side. Putting on the TV trying to stay up as late as possible hoping there would come a point where I would just pass out. But again every time I closed my eyes events of the last two days kept playing round and round my head, driving me mad.

The next thing I remember was suddenly waking up the clock said one thirty, looking around noticing the TV was playing to itself, both cats were lying next to me so close I couldn't move even if I wanted to. So looking up at the ceiling in the dark thinking of the last four years, trying to make sense of what had happened, was there a purpose to any of it? In 2006 as if it was yesterday, Dad becoming ill and facing the battle of his illness. Every two weeks travelling to the hospital for his chemotherapy treatment.

In 2007 I discovered a lump under my arm, back and forth to the hospital for tests, then to get an appointment at the Oncology Department. Automatic dread thinking the worse, especially with what happened to dad but thankfully the lump was not malignant. Then dad passing away and as if that wasn't enough both of Aaron's grandparents and his uncle lost their lives. Then to top it all in April 2009 Aaron's brain injury, so you could say I've had my fair share of horrendous luck.

My mind started to run away with itself my life just then seemed so uncertain, putting on some music praying this would calm me down taking away my fears. Anything to drown out the silence, nothing too morbid so playing everything I had by Linkin Park certainly not music to sooth the mind. Feeling myself drift off I remember Bonnie tapping my face with her paw I looked over at the clock, six thirty, "yes" I shouted punching the air, sleep had finally taken over.

Friday at last, to say it had been a long week is a bit of an understatement. Dragging my body slowly into the bathroom I stood under the shower for a while, hoping the memories of the last few days could be washed away. If only it was that simple. Something was driving me that day, hard to describe what that felt like but for some reason could not wait to get to the hospital. Aaron was having another scan, routine after this type of surgery or so I was told. Just hope it was good news.

It's funny what you notice when you're travelling, especially if you're not the one driving. Usually when you want to get somewhere in hurry cars appear from nowhere. Every traffic light seems to be against you. Passenger road rage takes over. Then when you get to your destination there are no parking spaces. That's what the journey felt like, once parked I made my way to the second floor in the lift, should take the stairs really but being afraid of heights and the fact the stairs are near glass windows with gaps in between the stairs made my legs turn to jelly. The long corridor from the lift to the NICU seemed endless with its shiny coating, was like walking a path into the unknown. Approaching reception we were greeted with a smile making our way to the relative's room it was a case now of waiting. Seemed busy today family's huddled together, sat in packs but everyone knowing we were all there for the same reason. Eyes watching and waiting for the door to open hoping you are the one that they call next. But for us it was two hours, the consultant came in not sure I wanted to hear what he had to say this time. My heart was pounding so loud I swear everyone could hear it. What if it was bad news not really prepared for that but when do you get ready for bad news.

He explained that there had been some brain damage to the left hand side of Aaron's head due to the size of the bleed he had sustained. Details taken from the medical report indicate that Aaron had an "extensive subarachnoid haemorrhage (SAH) with associated intra ventricular haemorrhage and a small intra cerebral clot in the left middle cerebral artery territory" to be precise. But to what extent that damage was is unknown that was until Aaron wakes up. All I heard was brain damage two words that screamed inside me, what does this mean? Does this mean he won't recognise me? What if this is how he is going to be? How could this have happened? Not much more to be done now until Monday so it had been decided to keep Aaron asleep and monitor him over the weekend. All I wanted to know was is he going to be ok? But no one could tell me.

I was so full of hope earlier, now I feel I am back where I started, that's it no expectations from now on, just take it one step at a time that way there will be no disappointment. It wasn't becoming a good day to make matters worse was the fear of dread sweeping over me knowing I had to go home to an empty house. It was a constant battle trying to unwind when all I wanted to do was relax and sleep. Seeing the doctor earlier that day to get signed off from work, having trouble looking after myself it was no good me being at work as well. All my strength had to be found to keep going so I could keep Aaron going, thinking of anybody else seemed too much to handle right now.

So here I am again home, why it is everything looks twice as bad at night? I remember it being about three o'clock in the morning. I sat on the stairs crying, no sobbing trying to work out why this has happened. I'm not religious but I do believe that everything happens for a reason, just what that reason is I have yet to work out. What little faith I had was lost that night, I also lost my way and part of myself. All I wanted to do was get into the car and drive, not sure where but anywhere seemed better than this. Without sounding selfish but I just don't think I could face life with Aaron as he was. Then the guilt set in, it wasn't his fault he was lying in a hospital bed fighting for his life, but on the other hand it wasn't my fault either. Fighting with myself was driving me insane for a while I really thought I was going mad. Maybe it was the fact I was totally exhausted that why I felt this way. Not thinking straight when all I needed was a good night's sleep. Although the doctor had prescribed me something to help me I just could not bring myself to take them, what if the phone rang and I didn't hear it? Looking out of the window into the black of the night, looking at the sky it seemed blacker than ever. Eventually the crying stopped, feeling a sense of release like the steam had been freed from a pressure cooker. Trying to think sensibly I knew I had to go back to bed, try to sleep and face what lie ahead the next day otherwise I would be no good to anyone, especially Aaron.

The next few days that followed were pretty much the same, Aaron's condition was stable the pneumonia was still not shifting so another swab was taken to see if the medication could be changed. With all this going on Aaron was also transferred to a rotating bed, I know what you're thinking you can imagine him going round like a chicken on a rotisserie, that thought had crossed my mind to. The reason for this was to help keep the lungs moving. Along with that there was also a concern as Aaron's temperature kept going up. To reduce this he was placed in bubble wrap with what looked like a large de-humidifier at the end of the bed. What a sight one minute the bed would vibrate it sounded like a washing machine on the spin cycle, then the bed would tilt from left to right. It was hard to see him in this state but I had to put my trust in the staff as they knew what they were doing.

During the course of the day one of the nurses decided to give Aaron a shave, watching him he looked so peaceful. Once she had cleared up the time had come to check his pupils she shone a light into his eyes, I remember her saying his eyes were like "sunflowers" all "bright and shining" letting us know he is still here. What a wonderful thing to say. On the same day doctors changed the lines in Aaron's neck and hands, bless him he had more holes in him than a colander. I'm quite squeamish when it comes to anything medical but I have a lot of respect for those who are dedicated into looking after the sick, especially to those who cannot do anything for themselves. It must be hard for any human to lose dignity, but when faced with being so incapacitated you trust others will try and give you back some of the decorum you once held.

Each day I would sit by his bed side knowing the time would come to leave, what made it more difficult was the not knowing. You imagine what has happened to others is automatically going to happen to Aaron. Something having to dismiss this from my mind, nothing was certain. Then as predicted I'd go home again feeling like I was on a constant treadmill. Days were rolling into one I started to get into a routine each day being the same as the last. Each night at home fight with myself to try to relax. The home that was full of life was now just a cold, empty shell with no life running through it. I missed Aaron mess, the noise and lights on everywhere, things that make life typical, that's what I craved the most and at that point I would give anything to have it back.

It's been just over a week since the injury and it was time to wake Aaron up again the pneumonia was slowly subsiding and his temperature now stable. So we waited and waited for him to come round, it seemed to take forever but eventually he opened his eyes, but there were no response signs at all which was of concern. There was this vacant look in his eyes a look I will never forget, being memorised trying to get him to look at me. Suddenly jumping out of my skin, his facial expression changed chewing on the pipe that was in his mouth but his eyes remained vacant. Standing there for a minute I watched for him to do it again. The nurse assigned to him that day started to carry out certain procedures, writing down stats but after a while you could see the oxygen levels dropped. The longer I was there the more I got used to how the machines worked and knew when something was not as it should be. In order to maintain his oxygen levels Aaron was put back under. By now I wasn't feeling so optimistic it looked like he'd never wake up, how much longer? I felt so deflated I was sure this time was going to be different. What happens if he doesn't respond at all? What if this is it?

The journey back home that night was very long, staring out of the window seeing my reflection in the glass trying to convince myself not to give up. Aaron was a fighter so until we knew what we were dealing with I could not give up either. The only trouble was my head and my heart were telling me two different things, do I cut my losses and run or do I stay and fight. It was down to me and me alone to decide what to do, it's not something to be taken lightly and I would not blame anyone in the same position to feel the same way. This is one of the hardest situations I have ever been in and throughout all of this I have followed my intuition. So far it's not let me down.

Back at home I phoned my mum for the first time since Aaron's injury. She was still on holiday but was trying to get home early, I told her not to as I was ok and being looked after the last thing I wanted was to worry her. I tried not to cry on the phone, just hearing her voice was enough when she told me everything will be alright a sense of calm overtook me. Just hearing her voice was all I needed. It sounded as though she was having a good time, which she deserved. I hung up and sobbed, not sure if it was because I missed mum and dad or if it was because of the day itself. In bed I closed my eyes and part of me wished I was a little girl again and my parents were there making everything better, the sense of feeling protected. How quickly life can become complicated when you grow up.

Early next morning I rang the hospital to be told Aaron was breathing on his own, from one day to the next what a difference, feeling euphoric and trying to forget what had happened the previous day and trying to look forward. The consultant was looking to operate later that day to fit a trachea into his throat, which would be easier for him when he wakes up. Surgery wasn't going to take long so before we knew he was back on the unit. Once settled it was time to reduce the sedation. With everything crossed this time I knew he was going to wake up. Eager to get to the hospital as I didn't want to miss this also I didn't want Aaron to be alone. Once there we discovered Aaron was awake, he'd been yawning and flexing his arms it was the most wonderful sight I'd seen in a while. After almost giving up any hope of him coming round to now seeing life slowly reappear was a moment to be cherished.

I can remember standing at his bedside holding his hand, speaking to him to see if he would make eye contact. It was like watching a child wake up and not quite knowing what to do. Checking to see if he recognised me, but I got nothing. My heart sank what if it was true that he has completely changed and does not know who he or even I am. It took all my strength not to cry. Over the next

48 hours Aaron continued to improve slowly. He wasn't responding much to commands, some of the tests I must admit seemed quite cruel but I know they had to be done. The nurse gave me instant reassurance, doing this every day made me trust them in whatever they had to do. There was very little or no response from Aaron's right side, which I was told was quite normal due to the size of the bleed on his left hand side, the question was, was it permanent? Praying that it wasn't the process begun now to try and repair him. I knew I could go home at night with the peace of mind that Aaron was being cared for 24/7. In the NICU each patient had a nurse allocated to them, watching every move like a guardian angel, making sure every detail was monitored and recorded. Having that responsibility of someone's life in your hands to me is a terrifying thought.

Slowly the nights were getting easier, after a good day followed a bad one it was learning how to deal with them. Aaron was in the best place they were doing all they could for him, the longer he was still alive the better his chances. All I had to deal with was getting through each day. Trying to convince myself that tomorrow was a new day no matter what has happened the plan was to look ahead. Sometimes it was easier said than done. Following day was my birthday, one I'm not looking forward to for the fact of being another year older, if I could have postponed I would have. Certainly not a day for celebration but one I will never forget in a hurry.

14<sup>th</sup> May 2009 not really in the mood that day, woke up not feeling too great, think the last few weeks were beginning to catch up with me. Dragging myself out of bed I showered, dressed and made my way downstairs. Cards were lying on the dining room table ready to be opened. It didn't feel right putting them up. The only thing I wanted was for Aaron to recover, nothing else mattered.

Was being picked up that day and whisked off early as friends had organised a birthday tea. My main focus was seeing Aaron this morning, just like every other morning. The journey to Oxford was like a ritual now, getting to know all the landmarks along the way. Starting to feel anxious before we've even got to Oxford, I think it's the thought of leaving early for the first time. For a split second I wanted time to stop so more moments could be spent with Aaron. Having second thoughts about leaving early the only problem with that was my lift to the hospital had to be home for a certain time. Feeling so guilty for not spending the day, what if he woke up and no one was with him? A constant emotion I would come to feel in the months ahead. Parking was a nightmare at John Radcliffe spending at least twenty minutes scouting for a space getting agitated as it was time wasted. The trip along the corridor seemed longer today. Nodding at the receptionist as we approached it was straight into the relative's room. There seems to be a lot of hanging about is this punishment for leaving early? Half an hour passed and I was pacing the room, the door opened and Aaron's nurse apologised for the wait as it had been one of those mornings tell me about it, having one myself.

As we followed her into the NICU I was approached by one of the other nurses and handed a card, how thoughtful it put a smile on my face at least. The closer I got to approaching Aaron's bed I could see a red rose had been placed across his arm, filled with embarrassment everyone started to look at me. Leaning over I kissed Aaron for a second he seemed to respond, thinking I'd imagined the nurse added "I saw that, he knows you're here" funny how they know how to say the right words at the right time. If only he would open his eyes a sign that he knows I was there. But for now I had to take what I could.

Aaron had been off the ventilator now all morning looking good so far, just before lunch the Physiotherapist came round they were looking to try and sit Aaron up for the first time. Unfortunately I could not be there to see it as it would be done during the patient's respite period, which was a time when there was no visiting. Thinking this would be done before I left it would be nice to take away some good news. So before I had the chance to grab a coffee I'd heard that Aaron managed to sit up for about five minutes with assistance even managed to lift his head which was a good sign. Feeling more positive now than when I arrived earlier. It was then time to leave, "already" was my reply "we've only been here a couple of hours" Reassuring me he would be fine, I left.

Day 22 a big day as Aaron was being moved from the NICU up to the Neuroscience ward upstairs, doctors were pleased with his progress and feel now he was ready to have rehabilitation and more stimulation. It was also a chance to see what his capabilities were since the brain injury. Filled with apprehension it was now time to be taken out of the comfort zone that we had been in for the last three weeks, knowing Aaron had 24 hour care was a saving grace. Aaron had been placed in this safe cocoon, now the real picture will develop. Being moved to this unknown place with different staff to try and build relationships with starting from scratch. The biggest worry for me was that he was being put into a room of his own, could he survive? Still was not communicating very well and very dependent on everyone. Not being able to move I was a little apprehensive to say the least. Not even sure yet that he even knew who I was let alone anyone else. On the other hand this was a step forward. If the doctors think it's time surly it was a risk worth taking. Seeing Aaron with all the wires and lines removed, apart from the feed drip and catheter made Aaron look quite normal. Along with my other concerns was that now he had been moved there were restrictions on visiting. Not quite sure how I was going to cope with that. The realization had not kicked in but I'm sure once it does panic again will take over.

Even when calling to check on him I found how much more difficult it was, getting through the phone would just ring at the other end. Not that It was any fault of the staff as they were too busy to just sit and answer the phone. This was just something I had to get used to. It was all good though because after a couple of day's doctors were looking to remove the trachea, but how soon would he be able to talk? It would be strange to hear Aaron voice after all this time, not really thought about if his speech had been affected. Once the trachea removed the speech and language therapist could work with Aaron more closely. It seemed by now that everything was moving quite quickly, so many different specialists, expert in their own field to advise from on what we were about to face.

Going home that night I was full of anxiety and optimism, convincing myself all will be ok. Aaron was slowly on his way back shouldn't be long now. Little did I know then how slow his recovery would be?

All the days that followed were an uphill trek. After the trachea was taken out Aaron did not speak. The consultant said it may take a couple of days as he would still have a sore throat. But after a week he was still not talking all we got were nods or shakes. It became difficult trying not to treat Aaron like a child when all his actions seemed to be in a child like manner. You could see the stubbornness within him taking over. Becoming like a disobedient child if he didn't get his own way. Trying to ascertain if he could remember my name or understand who I was? The only way to help was to bring in photos of family and friends and dot them around his room. To add to all this Aaron was becoming agitated with the feed line going up his nose, he would on many occasions attempt to pull it out and at one stage did. Knowing it should not be there made him worse. In the end he was made to wear giant padded mittens, what a sight you could see the frustration in his face it wasn't long before the determination took over to try and get them off. At least whilst visiting he didn't need to wear them. But you had to keep your eyes on him all the time. Before long It became apparent that the feed line had to be removed then Aaron was then put onto liquidised food. Looking at what he had to eat I think I preferred the line.

The weather was so lovely it was decided that we all needed a change of scenery, but it wasn't a simple as just getting up and going, preparations had to be made, firstly he had to be put into a wheelchair, for this he had to be hoisted up in a giant sheet and placed gently into the chair. This was the first time he had seen him out of bed since 28th April. I asked the staff if it would be ok to take Aaron outside for some fresh air, without hesitation they agreed it would be good for him, boosting his oxygen levels that had been fluctuating lately. I don't think we really appreciate how difficult it is pushing someone round in a wheelchair until you have to do it. The hike to the lift was enough suppose this would be another obstacle I'll have to overcome, depending on whether this was temporary or permanent. Once out the sun was beaming, Aaron started to squint the brightness of the light was putting a strain on his eyes plus the fact he hadn't seen much daylight for a while. Passing him a pair of sunglasses to wear it seemed a shame to hide his eyes away after we had only just started to enjoy them. Sitting in the hospital grounds feeling the sun warm on my face was a welcomed distraction, closing my eyes I imagined we were on a beach somewhere and none of this has happened. Then watching as Aaron's face caught the sun, getting his colour back was good to see. Seeing the inside of a hospital for so long you forget the outside world still exists. I then tempted him with an ice cream, watching him eat it giving him assistance to hold it as other people looked on. To be honest I thought this would bother him but he knew no different. With all the weight that Aaron had lost I was trying to get as much solid food in him for the liquidised food was so unappetizing he just wouldn't eat it.

Whilst basking in the sun my mind turned to the constant travelling and visits finding they eventually get you down. At one point I felt that if things were not going to improve I had to make decisions on what I was going to do. But knowing my mind was not in a good place I was in no position to make any rash decisions. Especially now that Aaron was out of the NICU and as I thought potentially out of danger. So the main priority was to make sure he was ok. For what would that make me if I abandoned him now? So I stayed.

# Chapter Three

## *On the move*

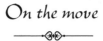

4<sup>th</sup> June 2009 today is the day that Aaron is on the move back to Kettering, totally unaware that this was happening when we arrived at Oxford that day. Not long after arriving I asked to speak to the doctor as concerns flashed in my mind. He's not ready to go back? He needs more time? What happens now? Whilst waiting I tried to convince myself it was for a good reason if not why are they making this decision? The doctor then entered the room explaining that they were pleased at this stage with Aaron's progress. Surgically they had done all they could for him the next step was expert rehabilitation, which Oxford could not offer. But how do we get that rehab? It had been decided so all that was left to do was pack all of Aaron's belongings with hope as well as apprehension. All that was left to do now was to wait for his ride back to Kettering. Aaron seemed blissfully unaware of what was happening, which in a way was no harm. By mid afternoon it was time to make a move, so once again hoisted up and placed on the ambulance bed he was wheeled downstairs. This time I got to travel back with Aaron in the ambulance with his parents following behind. Safely secure we set off, the journey was quite settled I actually think to some degree he enjoyed it. It's funny what you notice, the little things that no one else picks up on. To me I noticed since his admission to the ward he got into a habit of constantly holding paper tissues, this fascination and obsession with them took over. He'd sit for hours running it through his fingers, touching the end of his nose or simply just holding it like a comfort blanket. A look of contentment would appear on his face. As a silence fell in the ambulance I looked out of the window and reflected back on what had gone on so far, so much has happened in so little time, to think five weeks ago it could have been a different story.

As we approached Kettering, panic for me set in as the events of that first day came flooding back. A memory I feel will remain in my mind for a long time. Pulling up to the bay and once unloaded Aaron was taken to the old part of the hospital. My first impressions were not good the ward had eight beds in it, all of the other patients were a lot older than Aaron. The ward itself was really run down it was like stepping back in time. Looking around I thought I could not leave him here? Not being able to move or speak for himself, how was he going to cope? The other patients could not make out why Aaron would not speak although I explained to them the reasons I was not totally convinced they understood. What made it worse was now visiting was for one hour in the afternoon and one hour in the evening, that wasn't enough? Hoping his stay here was temporary, until a rehabilitation unit could be found. I was devastated having to leave him that night, I know no harm would come to him but no one at that stage knew exactly what he'd been through. If I could have stayed the night there I would have.

Back home I cried myself to sleep all what I had felt at the beginning was coming back up to the surface all I could think about was Aaron alone in a strange place not being able to ask for help if he needed it. How much more could I take? Could this get any worse, do I have the strength to carry on? Whilst lying there I contemplated calling hospital but did not want to appear obsessed. There was nothing I could do but accept the situation and keep going.

Patience was wearing thin the following day, eager to get to the hospital. Parking was a nightmare, it seemed as though everyone turned up at the same time. The lift took forever going to every other floor but the one I was on. Eventually turning the corner into the ward I took one look at Aaron his face said it all, lit up with a sense of relief if he could have spoken he would have said "get me out of here" "take me home" if only I could. Having a plan in mind to spend more time with him I wandered off to have a word with the ward sister the idea was to see if I could come in early to look after him hoping this would free up the nurses to do other things, the idea was welcomed and accepted with appreciation.

Another reason for going in to care for him was to make sure he had a familiar face with him for as long as he could. What made matters worse was that he was slowly becoming depressed which I'm told is common in brain injury. The doctor prescribed anti-depressants more pills, he was having problems taking the ones he was having as if it wasn't enough now he had depression to deal with, a battle on its own. Along with all that Aaron had to have regular injections to prevent blood clots, which had to be administered via the stomach and was known to sting the reason I know this was because as soon as the first one was given he said his first word, although he swore it was fantastic to hear.

Six days later Aaron was eventually moved to the High Dependency Ward (stroke ward). This unit was situated near the car park on the ground floor also newer than the one he just left. Being adapted more for Aaron's needs it laid my mind to rest. The atmosphere was totally different from the old ward I had a feeling Aaron may settle better. The staff appeared very welcoming and gave me a great deal of support over the next couple of weeks. I spent more hours here than at home. Arranging to come in and care for Aaron as visiting hours still applied as they did in the previous ward. By now the catheter had been removed due to him developing a urine infection. Unfortunately Aaron was still not in control of his bladder so needed constant help during the day as well as at night to change. At times my heart went out to him, all of the dignity he once had had now gone but thankfully he was oblivious to it. My role had now definitely changed from wife to full time carer. Giving far too much for far too long, at times I was finding there was nothing left to give.

During his time in the High Dependency Ward Aaron began to rebel, refusing to take his medication, not eat. It got to the point where the staff would wait for me to arrive to see if I could assist in some way by gentle persuasion. At meal times I would feed him the concept of holding a folk or spoon picking up food and transporting it to his mouth would not register. Crushing his medication and mixing it in his drink so he would at least take it without knowing, it seemed the only way he would take them. The sad thing was he acted more like a child than an adult, not one of the easiest tasks I've had to perform, especially when it involves a man you married and shared a life with. Aaron had lost about two stone, his clothes didn't fit him anymore but I suppose not being out of bed didn't help. His speech was still non-existent on the odd occasion he'd say "Yes" or "No" but nothing else. Little by little introducing different things to occupy his mind wasn't even sure if he could read. Up to this point it was trial and error to find out what to do as far as getting Aaron motivated. Playing DVD's setting up his IPod, which seemed to make him move to the music that was until he decided to eat the headphones. There's was no manual to follow telling you what to do or not to do at what stage, with brain injury everyone reacts differently. At least with a broken leg you know what's going to happen. For me that was the worst part of it all. I felt I was slowly losing my husband and a stranger was taking over but I had to carry on praying the old Aaron would somehow miraculously appear.

This particular day I arrived ready for the lunch run to find Aaron's bed needed changing, the nurses were stretched but it needed two of us to roll Aaron back and forth to change, not just him but the bed as well. I was run ragged by now I was washing clothes twice a day to try and keep up with his demands. Eventually assistance arrived, curtains were pulled around the bed and the process begun as it did many a time. The routine was now down to a fine art now and I knew exactly what to do. Instructions were given to Aaron on what we wanted him to do but knowing Aaron and how stubborn he could be didn't make it easy at times. On this occasion Aaron was being rolled towards the nurse when he muttered under his breath, I knew what he had said. Not sure if I was hearing things the nurse turned to me and said "did I just hear that". I turned to Aaron and asked him to repeat what he had just said, but as usual nothing.

18th June 2009. Not long after lunch had finished the Occupational Therapist came and managed to get Aaron sitting on the end of the bed. It took a great deal of work on their part as Aaron is over six foot and although he had lost two stone after being in bed since April he had no strength to do anything, plus the paralysis made it harder. All credit to Aaron though he tried to do most of the work which was good to see. It felt like there was real determination in what he had just achieved but it took what energy he had. Completely exhausted all he wanted to do then was sleep. For me I had chance to sit down and read for a while, quite a rarity these days. Knowing he'd sleep for about half an hour my thoughts turned to taking him outside later as the sun shone through the windows all my thoughts were on what to do for Aaron, none were for my benefit, for me I was at a complete loss.

Aaron woke up after about half an hour suggesting we go outside for some air was received with a smile. Walking round the ward looking for assistance to help get Aaron into a wheelchair the Physiotherapists came over. They had been contemplating taking Aaron to the gym at some point and as they had a free period there was no time like the present. Taking a slow stroll through the hospital grounds we headed to the gym, the idea was to see just what Aaron could do. Getting him up out of the chair they made him hold onto the parallel bars with me standing at the other end giving him encouragement. The two Physiotherapists stood either side of Aaron and with assistance got him to walk for the first time since his injury. I cannot tell you what I felt at that point but just watching someone you care for try and overcome such a huge obstacle, made my heart lift. Watching as he tried to put one foot in front of the other with such determination on his face. I could feel the tears roll down my face It then made me realise how much we do take for granted each day, when there are so many others suffering to do the simplest of tasks. Feeling elated and proud of what Aaron had so far achieved as he made his way towards me. When he was in arms reach I could wait no longer, wrapping my arms around his waist with such pride, seeing him looking down at me he probably wondered what all the fuss was about. Don't know about Aaron but after all that excitement I felt absolutely exhausted, feeling each step myself it was me that needed rest. Back on the ward and once settled in bed it was time for another nap. I rested my head on Aaron's bed as he slept, occasionally looking as he lay there thinking he was once the protector. A man who when he put his arms around you would make you feel safe. A man who was now lying in a hospital bed behaving in a childlike state having everything done for him, made my heart feel heavy. I watched him as his face twitched wondering what was going on in his head, knowing as he battles with his mind, he was slowly disappearing into a world I knew nothing about and probably never will a world I could not enter, feeling powerless to help all I could do was be there and support him in whatever way I could.

Not long after being back one of the doctors came to see me, he explained that Aaron's recovery is going to take a while anywhere from 6 months to possibly years. Although physically he may recover quickly, cognitively no time scale can be set. The doctor's words that day played on my mind this is an area I knew nothing about it felt that I was walking blind into the unknown. Plenty of food for thought needed. Leaving that night made me realise how precious life is and we should be grateful for what we have.

Being at home on my own was becoming a little easier although still not knowing exactly when Aaron would be coming home. The sooner specialist rehabilitation could be arranged the better. Not that the treatment Aaron had been given so far was to be criticized, but now he no longer needed the care of the hospital.

June 16th 2009 feeling nervous my first day back at work since Aaron's injury. Doing only four hours to start with, although nervous I was looking forward to another distraction something else to occupy my mind a chance to catch up with everyone. It was also the first day in my new role so new things to learn. The morning flew by it seemed as though I had been away for years not a couple of months. It took most of my time reading e-mails and being briefed on all the changes. So before I knew it I was in the car on my way to the hospital to do my other job getting ready for another day's battle wondering what mood Aaron was in today.

By now I was making decisions for both of us some days deciding what to wear was hard enough, let alone making life changing decisions for another person. It was down to me to sort everything out, becoming power of attorney for Aaron when normally we were both independent and used to making our own decisions. It was tough financially I was now the only one working, which was added pressure bills still needed to be paid. All of this, along with work and the hospital left little time for anything else.

It was good in a way to get back into a routine having work other than the hospital in my life. On 23th June Beechwood Rehabilitation Unit were coming to assess Aaron at Kettering. Hopefully not too long now before he was on the move. This time I was eager as this was hopefully the last journey before home, beginning now to see a light at the end of this very dark tunnel. It was about one before I got there, moving back the curtain I found him sat crossed leg in an arm chair looking quite relaxed. It was good to see him dressed and sitting instead of lying in bed, although the clothes he wore hung off him. Looking different now he'd lost all the weight, drawn in the face but not too gaunt. Taking one look at him you would be blissfully unaware of what was going on in his head. Waiting anxiously two people arrived from Beechwood firstly wandering about the unit before coming over to assess Aaron. Their aim was to ask him a series of questions and set simple tasks, like shaking hands, touching his nose. Some of which he responded to, other's there was nothing, not sure if it was that he did not understand or that he did not want to participate. He must have felt like a he was on display with everyone watching. The assessment lasted about 10 minutes as soon as it was over they shook Aaron's hand with the indication that they would be happy to take him. All that stood in the way now was waiting for a place, just hope we didn't have to wait too long.

Later that afternoon and feeling more confident we went to get some fresh air around the grounds with Aaron safely in the wheelchair. Another glorious day it's amazing what a bit of sun can do. Watching the world go by gazing at people come and go. Today had so far been a good day, enjoying the moment I sat smiling which I must admit had not been a regular occurrence just lately. Turning to look at Aaron I could see that the day had been a bit too much so we headed back. Safely back in the unit one of the nurses bounded over, smiling from ear to ear. They had just had a phone call from Beechwood to say that Aaron could be moved tomorrow, my first thought was to call work to see if I could get the day off so I could be there when Aaron moved. Turning a corner it felt like things were finally on the up. Travelling back home today felt different, a feeling of real optimism, could the worse be behind us?

It's been nearly two months now since Aaron's brain injury, up to now there has been good progress. But the obstacles to follow would test me beyond belief.

# Chapter Four

*The rehabilitation journey begins*

———◈◈———

2 4th June 2009-For the first time in a long while I didn't sleep too badly. I was woken by the sound of the phone, for a minute I thought I was dreaming. Turning over to look at the clock, it was nine thirty. Picking it up the voice on the other end was one of the nurses from Kettering hospital to say Aaron had just been collected and was on his way to Beechwood. I don't think she even had time to say goodbye, I quickly replaced the receiver and ran into the bathroom. Trying to judge how long it would take them to get from Kettering to Wellingborough I planned my getting ready down to the last minute. No knowing what to expect when I got to Beechwood as I had not been to see it before hand, I wanted Aaron to have someone there he knew when he arrived.

The advantage of Aaron moving here was that it was only 10-15 minutes from home, which was nothing compared to the trek to Oxford just two months ago. By the time I arrived found somewhere to park Aaron was already there. Beechwood Rehabilitation Unit is on the grounds of Isebrook Hospital, Wellingborough, Northamptonshire. The unit is on one level with what looked like flats above. It has been purpose built with a spacious reception, lounge/dining area, with a large activity/therapy room. It has ten rooms with five self contained flats all with en-suites. The main purpose of the unit is to provide high quality rehabilitation, for adults who have problems neurologically, ranging from strokes, multiple Sclerosis and acute brain injury to anyone suffering from musculoskeletal problems such as arthritis or severe back pain.

The sense of the place felt right and I knew and hoped Aaron would settle here for as long as it took. It's like anywhere new when you go for the first time, curiosity takes over and it wasn't long before I found my way around. We were greeted in reception by staff, who seemed pleasant and welcoming offering assistance straight away. Aaron was placed in a room of his own, smaller than the one at John Radcliffe less clinical and more comfortable. He had a large window and door leading out to a tiny garden. This was situated at the front of the unit so you could see the comings and goings. I felt a sense of calm about the place and hoped Aaron wouldn't take long to adjust. The world to him must be confusing enough without being transported from one place to another, not knowing where you are going and why you are being sent there. Then with me arriving then leaving unable to explain in words that he understands why he has to stay. When even doing the simplest task seem like a mammoth ordeal. A sense of feeling trapped like a caged animal with only one thought and that is to be free.

The doctor was due to see Aaron later in the day to welcome and examine him, the move didn't seem to have too much of an impact on him, but it was hard to say as he still would not speak. After unpacking he was settled in bed. It was then he attempted to get out I could see the frustration in his face when his efforts failed. Why can't I do this? I began to worry what if he tried to get up in the night and no one was about? At least in Oxford and Kettering there were sides on the bed, here there were none. The staff reassured me that he would be fine. With no 24 hour care this is when I felt the real fight starts.

After an hour it was nice to see a friendly face, our friend Michelle and her daughter Hannah aged two turned up, Michelle had been there since day one so she knew how far Aaron had come. With Michelle being there I hoped another face this would give him something else to focus on. Aaron had not seen Hannah since the injury, it was interesting to see how he reacted to her, I asked him if he knew who she was he nodded and smiled. She shuffled behind her mother's legs all shy and timid, playing peek-a-boo with him until she was comfortable in the surroundings.

Five minutes into their visit and knowing they were staying a while gave me a chance to quickly go back home to pick up a few more clothes for Aaron, that's if I could find clothes to fit him now with all the weight he has lost, looks like shopping was next on my list. Visiting times were more flexible so it would fit in around work. It would also give me more time, one thing that would become a blessing to me later on especially now the travelling had been greatly reduced. Things I thought were beginning to find their feet a little. I called his parent's to let them know he had moved and what times visiting were. Slowly we could introduce a scheduled visiting time so he did not have too many visitors at once.

The rest of the day went without any hitches. Aaron was now on solid food which in itself was a big step at least he was eating more now. However some of the options on the menu Aaron would not eat. I put together a list of likes and dislikes to assist staff when I was not there. Trying to stay positive I spoke to him trying to get him to understand why he had to be there, hoping that home was the next step. Whether he acknowledged just what I had said was unknown. The plan for tomorrow was that the Physiotherapists were coming along to assess Aaron, the sooner he starts his rehabilitation the better. My aim was to have as much input as allowed so that I could learn as well. My plan was to go back to work the next day and finish at lunch time, call at home first then straight to Beechwood for the rest of the day. Any help that I could give made me feel as though I was doing something at least.

I could see the day had taken its toll on Aaron so I decided to leave sitting on the bed Aaron gently placed his head upon my shoulder. I stroked his hair, my heartfelt heavy and my thoughts turned to wonder if he will ever get through this. Even more so would I get through it? I got up and as I walked out I saw the sadness in his eyes as I could see he wanted me to take him home. It took all my strength just to walk out and not look back.

I cried all the way home, where am I going to find the strength to do this? How long is it going to take before Aaron gets back to normal? But what is normal? All I want is my life back is that too much to ask for? I knew that night before I got into bed I wasn't going to get much sleep my mind just would not switch off. The thought of Aaron trying to get out of bed was a concern and if he did succeed would he injure himself? I felt really low a constant feeling I'd been having recently. Why am I trying to re live what has happened? Nothing I can do will change it? All I had to do was let's see what happens be it good or bad. Surely things cannot get any worse can they?

25th June 2009, I was working till 1130hrs this would be a regular routine for me for the next few weeks. One good thing was that I had no calls during the night which was a blessing. Or was it that they were waiting for me to arrive and speak to me in person. If you have not noticed by now I tend to worry it's a trait with me, always has been. But recently I have learnt to let it subside a little for my own sanity more than anything.

Work was becoming a very welcomed distraction by now, although my thoughts were constantly on Aaron, work became my saving grace it was what I needed at that point, giving me a sense of purpose. Some of my colleagues are good friends out of work as well as in so no matter how bad my day is or how I am feeling when I turn up, they are there to lend a shoulder. I do on the other hand try and maintain a professional approach to work by keeping my feeling under control, sometimes easier said than done. The mornings at work go quickly I am kept busy within my new role. So before long it's time to leave to start my other full time job.

Now that I didn't have to travel so far I felt less tired which was a bonus as I could focus more on helping to get Aaron through this difficult period. I learnt on my arrival to Beechwood that Aaron had been given a shower, he was none too pleased about it though as he had to be wheeled into the bathroom and washed by two carers as he did not have the ability to do it himself. Frustration and confusion were to play a big part in the rehabilitation process. A process that Aaron was not pleased at joining in with. I went to his room to find it empty, I wandered about to find him in the gym where the Physiotherapists were trying to get him to use the parallel bars. I stood back and watched. How can a man, who was full of life, be reduced to not being able to do anything for himself in such a short space of time? I don't think we fully understand and appreciate how powerful the brain can be. I stood there for about five minutes I could see he'd had enough. Another side affect of brain injury is that fatigue takes over you so quickly and before long all Aaron wanted to do was go back to his room and get into bed. After a rest maybe he would be up for going out to get some fresh air. This was still all new to me and I didn't know what to do, what to say, walking blind learning as I go along, making mistakes. Following advice from staff was all I had. Was I hoping for too much too soon? Is what I'm feeling normal?

It was getting to the stage again where Aaron was refusing to take his medication, he was not the best at taking tablets before his injury so why should now be any different. It was bad enough him having to take them but not knowing why he had to take them I think I would have been a little unwilling. I found that he would only take them if I gave them to him so it was agreed with staff that they would wait till I arrived then gave the medication to me. My role as a carer was taking over my role as a wife, I'd forgotten what that side of our relationship was like. Even to this day I haven't yet got the role back full time. I have this man who is like a stranger to me, to look after in this child like state him having someone to depend on. I think his mother felt a little left out as this should be her role. Aaron did not adapt well to other people so I felt the pressure more, not that I minded but it was hard work. I can understand why loved ones and family give up. Your whole time is given to this person with nothing in return. Not that the fault lies with the sufferer they don't know what time or day of the week it is let alone saying thank you. It's not a selfish act on their part, but there are times when a feeling of resentment sets in.

When it's just you there the situation really hits home that this is your life, like it or not. Family and friends go home with lives of their own to lead, not really having that much impact on yours. They are still able to go out, have holidays do all the things you use to do before brain injury. Thinking one day we will do all those things again. My life was on hold until who knows, that's when doing the simplest of tasks like going out for a meal were impossible with Aaron the way he was. I also felt that I could not do those things without him, why should I go out when he was stuck in this indeterminate state. This is when the guilt set in. It's easy for people to say "you have to look after you" which at that point I had no interest in. Until you are placed in a position like this or any life changing role no one can tell you what to do. Not wanting to sound the victim here far from it, this is to try and explain to others in a similar situation that you are not alone, the feeling of no hope and loss are normal. It's only been in the last few months that I have not been so hard on myself and it does get easier with time. I feel more confident about the future and trying to stay positive, trying to install this into Aaron as well. It was hard as Aaron got depressed. Keeping his mood up was a task but with a bit of luck the medication would soon help him.

The next few days that followed not much progress took place, one good thing blew me away was when Aaron stood up for the first time on his feet, with support mind you. It was a wonderful feeling just to put my arms around him. At that point I didn't realise just how much weight he had lost, it felt like I was supporting a fragile figurine, daring not hold too tight just in case he snapped. This was a giant step forward to how he was a few weeks ago, lying paralysed not knowing if he would be able to move at all.

The weekend was upon us, the first one at Beechwood a few more visitors were expected today, although too many at once had already proved to be too much for him to handle. Noticing he was speaking a little more now made it easier, some words made sense other times he would go back to whispering and made no sense at all? The morning had been hectic with 3-4 people at once, most of the time Aaron sat confused just looking whilst they chatted away to him. It must have been hard for the visitors not knowing what to say, how to say it, do we speak normally to him? was one comment I got. By the afternoon peace had finally descended, it was a beautiful day all I craved for was some quality time with Aaron, time that I had not been able to have on my own since his injury. The idea was to go out across the road to the park, not too far just In case we needed to get back. I asked him where he wanted to go he replied "take me to Asda" he really knew how to treat a girl and show her a good time. What struck me most was the fact he just came straight out with it, word perfect. The thought of a supermarket on a Saturday afternoon didn't really appeal to me and to be honest it probably would have made him anxious and me very uneasy. So the park it was after getting into the wheelchair we headed out, the path leading there was uneven so by the time we got to the entrance and after pushing the wheelchair it felt like I had completed a half marathon. Being reasonably quiet I sat for a bit. It felt strange it just being the two of us and no one else about. Sitting in silence listening to the birds and children in the background playing, it was nice to finally have some peace amongst all the chaos that had occurred.

Drifting off into our own worlds fifteen minutes had passed when I looked over at Aaron asking if he'd had enough, he nodded in response to my question. I think he felt quite vulnerable out in the open knowing he could not do anything. Back in the unit I got him settled in bed once more putting on a DVD he eventually fell asleep. Everything Aaron did took so much effort, thinking back to how he was before the injury makes you shake your head in disbelief. But surely things from now on can only improve with time? As evening fell I looked back on the day a good one considering. When it came for me to leave I told him I would be back in tomorrow morning, now I was going home to feed the cats and sort out the washing, exciting life I was leading. I remember him saying "why do you have to do that" trying to explain to him he then put his arms around me it felt he wasn't going to let me go leaving him got harder each night. But for now there was nothing I could do, he was being looked after by people who knew about this, it was Aaron that had to be put first not me.

One thing I have noticed throughout this though, stuck in this nightmare time comes and goes. I keep reflecting back and comparing stages that Aaron has gone through. Even though it's now been over two months it feels like an eternity, so much has happened in a short space of time there have been moments when everything else is moving at a fast pace but I'm moving in slow motion. Clock watching has become part of the norm everything seems to revolve around time. What time is his next medication? How long before dinner? What time frame before he can come home? It's as though if the stages have a time frame the recovery won't seem so long. Looking at it on the other hand when you are told he will be home in September it seems to give a purpose to it all, a goal to work towards.

Aaron had been at Beechwood now for a week, doctor was due to do his weekly round. Being as though it was his first visit I wanted to be there so I had an idea what they were expecting from Aaron. Waiting with anticipation the doctor arrived, shook his hand and began the task of asking him a series of questions. It's very hard trying to keep quiet and not to answer for him but no matter what Aaron's replied I knew I had to just stand there. I remember the doctor asking Aaron to pass him a grape that was lying in the fruit bowl on his table. It was amusing to see him pick one, slowly aim it towards the doctor then as quick as anything put it in his own mouth. A sense of humour just what I'd been waiting for, that glimmer of wittiness that I longed to see was slowly peering through. After his action a grin appeared over his face, I had to laugh well he nearly got it right. After about ten minutes the doctor left after deciding to start and reduce the medication. Although he was still at risk of having an epileptic fit this was a good sign as the medication could have an impact on his memory and the ability to communicate better. "Could this be the start of him getting better" I thought? Once the doctor left Aaron had a shower it was a little strange as we found that he was becoming susceptible to water. He didn't cry out on pain but the look on his face indicated he wasn't happy. It was difficult as he could not explain why or how it felt. I was told that this was sometimes normal, not everyone experience this sensation with water but it can happen. Nothing else like clothes or touch seemed to bother him. I don't think it helped him not being able to shower himself, a loss of dignity and pride on his behalf.

As the menus at Beechwood did not always suit Aaron's taste I decided to go and get one of his favourite fast foods, just to see if his likes and dislikes had changed in anyway, plus I could eat with him. It had been a while since we last ate together, trying to make the surroundings a little more cosy we made the best of the situation, it was good to see him eat the majority of the food. It was interesting watching him, using mainly his fingers wasn't too bad, when it came to using cutlery he would often miss his mouth, but at least he was trying. Cutting food up was also a problem for him at the moment, so I did that for him. It was good to see him eating solid food after the weeks of him trying to digest liquidised food. Making the most of the evening I surprised him with music and comedy trying to make this evening as normal as I could. Seeing him laugh made everything seem un-important but before long reality hit and Aaron wanted to go bed, making sure he had what he needed I stayed a while.

I was finding I needed a lot of patience and tolerance with Aaron as each day passed it's not easy caring for a man who when you met and married had an aura about him, he was the protector I could rely and lean on whenever I required it. Now he is the one that needs the protection. This vulnerable guy displaying child like attributes who if was to be put back in society I believe would find it hard to cope and I believe we would not be together today. Wanting him to snap out of whatever was keeping him prisoner in his head, if only it was that easy. Maybe he would wake up one morning and all would be ok, miracles do happen. Or maybe it was just wishful thinking on my part.

It was becoming obvious as time went on that Aaron was not being very cooperative when it came to his rehabilitation. It was very difficult trying to describe to someone who has suffered a brain injury why it is important to do the simplest of tasks. When according to them they are ok. This was the case with Aaron it didn't help him being stubborn and argumentative, a feature that was to following in the fore coming months. He became very selective early on which members of staff he liked and those he didn't, he was displaying more swearing than normal and believe me before his injury he could swear, but for some reason it's been magnified. Feeling embarrassed each time he was rude I apologised more times than I can remember. The staff explained that they'd heard it on many occasions. People who suffered brain injury who never use to swear suddenly have this desire to do so. Every time I would visit there was not a moment that passed when you wouldn't hear someone somewhere swear.

1st July 2009 I attempted to give Aaron a shave today which would have gone ok if he sat still and did not moan all the time. His hair had been cut for the first time since April he was starting to look like his old self. If no one knew any better you'd be unaware of the torment that was going on in his head. Again another disadvantage of this "hidden disability" The weather was so hot today I tried to get him outside as much as I could a bit of sun did him the world of good, staying in was becoming hard. Trying to find things to keep Aaron occupied was a tall order in itself, the rehabilitation was not regular so before long he was starting to get bored.

I was trying to catch up with the Occupational Therapist (OT) and Physiotherapists (PT) to obtain feedback on sessions Aaron did attend, not a lot of consistency was the general feel but I'm hopeful that this will improve. Aaron was managing a couple of steps, with support and they were looking to progress Aaron onto a frame and for him to stop using the wheelchair altogether. His mood swings were up and down some days he wouldn't speak just nods and shakes. The dining room at Beechwood was where the resident's had to go for lunch and dinner. At times Aaron would not stay down there because it was too noisy, that seemed to be another issue with him. So every now and then he was allowed to eat in his room. Knowing he could do this made it more difficult getting him to the dining room. There are times when I find myself just looking at Aaron feeling sorry for him being in this position, not pity or sympathy just trying to get my head around as to why it's ended up like this. I've wanted to trade places with him on many occasions, knowing he's got to learn everything and I mean everything all over again. It's easy for us to take what we do for granted, things like making a hot drink, getting dressed in a morning, everyday jobs that we don't have to give a second thought to. Sitting by his bed he took hold of my hand and pulled of my wedding ring, looking and playing with it. I asked him if he knew what it was all I got was a nod. The action was like a curious child exploring for the first time.

It's sad to think that once we have grown up and have learnt all the basics in life, to then have an injury or illness that means having to learn everything from scratch does not feel right. Second time around seems to be harder to cope with especially as we get older. As a child your parents are there to protect and teach you right from wrong. Learning to walk again later in life takes more effort and not everyone has someone to encourage or protect them. Watching a loved one go through the torment and anguish when all you can do is watch. Yes you're there to support and give that little extra push but that sometimes isn't enough. Usually all the sympathy and help revolves around the sufferer but what about those left behind. From a wife or husband to other family members who not only have to deal with the trauma of what has happened. But to carry on with everyday life, holding down a job, making sure the family unit is kept intact finances are being kept up to date. So in all of this what about us?

Having and living with brain injury can be a lonely existence especially for a wife or husband of a sufferer. Before brain injury you share your life with this person, getting to know them, taking on their good as well as bad habits. But when brain injury strikes it's like they become a complete stranger. There in a shell with the real person fighting to get out. Having their brain dictating what they can and cannot do. The worse point I found with Aaron in the beginning was him not showing any emotion or compassion. All you crave is for them to hold you and tell you it's going to be ok. Sure having family and friends around for support helps but the loneliness you feel at night on your own was sometimes hard to bare. The longing for someone, knowing that it is not reciprocated fills you with slight resentment, not that it's their fault. This is when feelings change and the longer the injury goes on the harder it is not to feel it. You start to think if I hang around long enough will I ever get back what I had with this person? As recovery continues some sufferers make progress with this, personalities can change, this can be for the better or worse. With Aaron his aggression and patience have been heightened since his brain injury, to him he feels as though he is exactly the same as before and although to a certain degree he is, however there are moments when he has a "Jekyll & Hyde" side. It may only be for a couple of minutes but it's enough to make you feel uneasy. If he is at home at the time the situation can be challenged but when out in the community it makes the situation slightly more uncomfortable. With other people not knowing about his injury this is when he becomes vulnerable. Not knowing how long his recovery is going to take I'm hoping that he will adapt and become more tolerable.

It's the weekend again looking forward to it, my brother and his family are coming to see Aaron. They were bringing with them my new nephew Charlie, whom I have not seen since he was born just 3 weeks prior. Hoping this would give Aaron the incentive to get up, showered and dressed. They were due to arrive just after lunch, my brother was a little apprehensive not sure what to expect as he had not seen Aaron since the day of his injury, lying flat in the A&E connected to wires before he was transported to Oxford. Then with all the drama of the baby arriving he didn't have time to visit, which I understood. When they turned up Aaron was still in the dining room finishing his lunch this gave me time to fill them in on what to expect and if it got too much for them I would understand if they wanted to leave early.

I wheeled Aaron back to his room, he smiled at them all, a good start. But it was my other nephew Ben who was 5 that I noticed. He didn't quite know what to make of it, he'd seen Aaron as this strong man who was always joking about and who played with him. To see him now in a wheelchair hardly speaking looking gaunt due to the weight loss must have to him seemed upsetting. Keeping the mood and spirits up I suggested we all go outside, until it started to rain. Aaron's room was not adapted to take a large crowd so before long the kids were getting restless, which in turn agitated Aaron. Charlie had been fed and was now asleep. Aaron too wanted to lie down my brother took the other two down to the dining room for a breather. Sue (my sister in law) and I stayed with Aaron along with the baby. Out of curiosity Charlie was placed on Aaron's chest as he lay there, cradling him with such tenderness I felt a lump appear in my throat. It was as if he knew what to do straight away, how delicate the baby was and how he was to be handled. Lying there wrapping his arms around Charlie to protect this precious gift that had been given to him. It was a wonderful sight indeed.

A couple of hours had flown by and before long I was waving the family off, it was good to see them we have always been close, even more so since dad had died. Wandering back into his room I looked over to see him yawn, the day had worn him out. Deciding to leave earlier than normal which in a way didn't feel right but it gave me time to myself which was something that night I craved.

It was a couple of days later that Aaron was put onto a walking frame the wheelchair became surplus to requirements. It was going to be a lot easier not pushing him around also it would make Aaron work harder on his walking. It became apparent that now he found this new independent way of getting about there was no stopping him. He could wander off around the unit, watching him you could see physically he was getting stronger as each day but cognitively the fog was still very thick and as yet had not caught up with his body. Not knowing your own mind is something you cannot imagine, many times Aaron has said to me "you don't know what it's like" and no I don't. I cannot begin to imagine the torment felt, knowing that you are capable of doing certain things but your mind won't let you. The frustration and anguish, for example on his walk about he would wander into other resident's room which was not allowed. It was then when I tried to get him out and go somewhere else he would get irritated with me, which then made me angry thinking "why are you shouting at me" feeling I could do nothing right. Trouble was I had to let it go over my head, he didn't mean it they always say you hurt the ones you love. When you are tired, feeling low trying your best to care for someone and all they do is start shouting at you, there is only so much you can take. To Aaron though the things he was doing were perfectly normal. Then when I challenged him telling him that what he was doing wasn't right, he would swear at me which made him even more determined to do it and asking "why" a word that would become quite frequent.

Aaron was becoming more curious along with that came more care, he was like a child pushing your buttons seeing how far he could go before getting told off. At least when he was bed ridden he was easier to deal with, (not that I wish he was back there). This was all good recovery but sometimes a little too fast. Regular meetings were held at Beechwood with me and staff to discuss Aaron's progress and how we could move forward. The plan was to have Aaron home in September with 24 hour care although there was a lot of work to do it seemed the right move. A home visit would be required to make sure the house was suitable to see if any changes needed to be done before hand. Once he was home the recovery won't seem too bad. The rehab continued and I was getting in a routine counting down the days, didn't really think about how it was going to be when he came home I just wanted him there.

Every day I'd find Aaron would achieve something or maybe it was me hoping he'd accomplish more. Dressing himself was becoming more frequent, extra steps with his walking, things that amazed me, things I'd thought he'd never do again. What stuck in my mind the most was shoe laces, the first time Aaron put on his trainers he did the laces up without giving it a second thought, yet other tasks like showering were still a problem for him. Communication between us varied from day to day depending on what mood he was in. I never knew until I arrived what to expect. The medication that Aaron was taking at the time was still being reduced, maybe that could have suppressed his communication.

The frame Aaron was using got him everywhere he was becoming quite quick with it, the Occupational Therapist was looking to progress with sticks, a little more difficult more balance required on Aaron's part. His sessions in the gym on the balance ball were going to have to come into play. His standing and sitting were all improving all good steps for when he comes home. I was so proud of what Aaron had achieved but I knew there was a long way to go. Being at the unit was a full time job, leaving there I'd come home shattered there was little time left for anything else. Don't get me wrong the busier I was the better, It was my way of coping I think if I'd have slowed down or stopped I would have crumbled.

Car transportation was the next step for Aaron a joint process that I would assist in with the Occupational Therapists. This enabled Aaron to get in and out of a vehicle without causing more injury to him. We did try earlier on when he was still in the wheelchair but that was a major operation in itself that I'm sure with practice could have been mastered. But now with him being more mobile the process was a lot easier. At least it was something else I could do. Take him for rides in the car to stop him getting bored. The only problem in that was he thought he was driving, giving me directions, if I took a wrong turn he would get mad with me. We would end up having rows in the car I would then take him back to Beechwood. I had an idea about driving him to Rushden to see if he remembered any of it. Whether I did right or not I drove him up the road and asked him if he knew who lived at the house I pointed out, he nodded.

One good thing though he didn't make any attempt to get out of the car or asked to go in. Trips in the car became regular I thought it would do him good to get him out and about. Sometimes we would go round to friends but only for a few minutes. Giving him a sense of regularity but also being cautious in case he would not go back.

His cognitive state was starting to change and along with this came more mischievous antics, blocking toilets became a daily ritual. I can say that most days when I turned the staff would say "he'd blocked another one" remembering one evening after dinner going to find his door shut. I went in to find the bathroom door closed as well. On shouting his name I'd opened it to find Aaron standing there naked apart from socks putting items down the toilet. When I asked him what he was doing he replied "having a wash" It was sad to see, slowly managing to coax him back into the room and helping to get him dressed before his parents arrived.

Rehabilitation was only done about an hour a day Aaron had time on his hands, soon boredom took over and he began to pack all of his belongings and place them at the front door. He probably thought if I'm not doing anything here, let me go home. His room was a bare as when we first arrived, each time he said he was coming home and each time telling him not just yet was starting to wear thin. This process carried on every day from then on. It got to the stage when I would take something home with me so he'd have less to pack. The task was to keep him occupied as much as possible, although it was difficult me not being there until the afternoon. His resilience to comply with any form of rehab was getting difficult he would not partake in anything. A new strategy was called for. His timetable was adjusted so that his rehab would be carried out when I was there, hoping I could encourage him to join in. For a while it worked

Basically telling him that if he didn't do this he would not come home. Riddled with guilt he became angry with me but I had to be cruel to be kind for his own good no matter how much it was killing me.

The next afternoon Aaron had to get to grips with making hot drinks, this was a task that he had tried but with a lot of support. I think it was the remembering the process for him, so many bits to recollect. The planning and sequencing along with the ability to retain information would prove to be Aaron's biggest obstacle limiting his capabilities. This was a task that with endless practice he would eventually master. From him at the beginning when all he could do was to stare at the kettle trying to figure out what to do. The process became like a major operation to you and me not a second thought is taken when doing this. I could see the concentration and determination in his face the OT was prompting him most of the time. I think he wanted to prove to us and himself that he could do it.

We were approaching the end of another day at Beechwood just over a month to go before Aaron comes home. His communication skills were still improving, his physical appearance was getting better day by day. But it was his heightened cognitive state was becoming more demanding and unpredictable. There was times when I wished he was not as mobile as he was at least with him being confined to bed more I could keep a better eye on him. There seems to be more confusion on Aaron's part, his understanding of why he was there, no insight what so ever into his injury. That then presented a problem as he could not tell you what he was thinking or wanted.

24th July 2009 not having a good day today took the day off work. One reason was to re charge my batteries, try to rest for a few extra hours. Sometimes just having the space to have a dam good cry was all it took. There was no need calling beforehand to see how Aaron was. I knew if there was a problem they would call me. Looking at me on the outside strong and confident but on the inside every part of my being has been battered. Didn't go to Beechwood any earlier felt I needed time for me. When I did turn up one of the nurse told me that Aaron had had a fall during the night. Not sure how it happened but he was ok, although he has sustained a bruise at the base of his spine but no other injuries. I bet he tried to get up during the night and fell. When I asked him about it but he couldn't remember. He had already been checked out by the doctor just for peace of mind.

Just then the Physiotherapist walked in and suggested today's session was Aaron overcoming a flight of stairs. This was one not to be missed, giving him gentle persuasion on why he needed to go. The session would take place in the hospital itself. In order to get there Aaron would have to walk or be pushed in the wheelchair. The corridor was deserted, my role was to stand and observe whilst the two physio's stood either side of Aaron supporting his arms, guiding him. He listened to the instructions given and with each step took a smile would appear on his face. With each step made a chance for him to catch his breath. What a magnificent sight I was witnessing. All credit to him the session took nearly an hour but he managed going both up and back down.

Leaving him had not got any easier the thought of still going home to an empty house each night filled me with anxiety. The thought of going out and "having a good time" still did not feel the right thing to do whilst Aaron was still struggling. I know I needed a life to but what life the life I had had been taken from me without question so the last thing I wanted to do was enjoy myself. But how quickly you adapt and how life changes with time, although Aaron is still recovery I enjoy going out with friends and yes have a laugh.

Aaron was now going for walks out of the unit using a stick. However he was blissfully unaware of the dangers that lurked. Staff followed to try to persuade him back but he would become agitated and start shouting at them. The concern was him getting out and no one seeing him. Beechwood was not a secure unit and although everyone was doing their best they could not watch him all the time.

4th August 2009 a day when everything changed. I was at work as usual when my mobile rang as soon as I saw the number my heart sank. Looking up it was eleven o'clock. The receptionist from Beechwood had been told to call me, this morning Aaron had packed all his belongings became agitated and took off out of the unit. He was followed by one of the nurses claiming he was going. Panic set in I knew I had to leave heaven knows what he could do. It was going to take me at least forty minutes to get there all they had to do was pacify him until I arrived. I can't even remember the journey telling them to call me if the situation got any worse, not sure what I was going to do if it did. Thankfully traffic was light before long I was pulling into the road leading to the hospital. In the distance I could see Aaron attempting to climb a wire fence to get out onto the road. I stopped on the side of the road opposite Aaron got out and in a calm voice asked him what he was doing. I could see thrown over the fence already was his wash bag and a DVD, nothing else. He told me he was going home, trying with all my being to get him to come down from the fence he would not budge, I then drove round into the car park so he could get into the car. At least in there he would be safe, the nurse was stood back as Aaron just kept swearing at him. Not to make the situation any worse I asked the nurse to leave as I would try and get him in the car. It was now just the two of us he refused to move, I pleaded with him and eventually he came down to the safety of the car. Driving back towards the unit Aaron still angry said "I'm not going back in there" Switching off the ignition, I got out of the car, locked it and went in to talk to staff. They told me that if I had not have shown when I did they were going to call the police to get Aaron sectioned for his own safety. I could not let this happen surely there is another solution? Popping back outside to the car to see if Aaron was ok still filled with rage and hostility for the first time he scared me, just what would he capable of in this state of mind? He was still refusing to move I was at my wits end. The doctor had been called to try and see if he could prescribe something to calm him down. The likelihood of him remaining at Beechwood was limited they were not set up to deal with this level of cognitive state. Aaron needed a more secure unit to keep him and other's safe. Where had all this come from? Were the sign's there but just not being picked up? Has this been building up since he could walk? Was it a sign when he started to pack up all his belonging that he was going to attempt to leave? Could I have prevented this? I called his parents as I felt some of the responsibility could be put onto someone else close to him, maybe they could try and talk to him, stay with him until something could be resolved.

Phone calls were being made to other rehabilitation units for them to come and assess Aaron to see if they could meet his needs. At least three assessments were to be carried out from three separate units. Surely this would take too long time at present wasn't on our side.

Aaron had calmed down a little but he was adamant he was not staying here any longer. The question was how long was this process going to take? With short notice two rehabilitation units agreed to see Aaron today but no decision could be made until the third had been done. Becoming anxious myself I had the idea of someone being with Aaron round the clock to keep an eye on him just in case a repeat of earlier occurred. Arrangements were made with family and friends to take it in turns until other actions could be taken.

One of the assessments was carried out by Oakleaf Care they are based in Hartwell Northants. The idea was to speak to Aaron, ask him questions find out if they could help. Two members of staff arrived they spoke to Beechwood first. We sat anxiously in reception waiting to be called, I felt sick to my stomach. Aaron knew something was happening and I did tell him that he would probably be moved shortly, he replied "good"

I have never felt so tense, it was like applying for a job and this was the interview. My main concern was Aaron hoping he would to make a good impression and not become agitated. It was explained to us what Oakleaf Care was all about and what they could offer Aaron. This was just what Aaron needed a structure, routine and most of all to be safe. Oakleaf was more of a secure unit than Beechwood, the residents had the freedom to wander the grounds. The main doors were always locked and if they weren't and a resident tried to get out, alarms would sound. My mind had been made up then realising the other two assessments needed to be carried out first. Once all three had been completed, it was then down to the relevant unit to make the choice on whether Aaron was suited to their type of rehabilitation This day was not getting any easier I needed a break but felt I could not go anywhere just in case Aaron wanted to come. I could feel the fight in me subside, as though I had already given up. But I had to keep going if only for Aaron's sake. My thoughts turned to night ahead if I had my way I would have stayed all night. But staff reassured me they would keep an eye on him. By late afternoon there were enough of us there to give me chance to slip away for a while. As I got into the car, Aaron spotted me, dashing he got in beside me saying he was coming. Without hesitation I could have driven off with him there, but I knew I couldn't the trouble was he didn't understand why. I sat behind the wheel feeling myself break down seeing me like that I think made him change his mind because within seconds he got out of the car and wandered back into the unit. By then I didn't want to leave but after some gentle persuasion by staff I came away I was absolutely exhausted but somehow from somewhere I found the strength to carry on.

When I returned he was tucked up in bed chatting to his two mates claiming he would stay tonight but adamant he was leaving tomorrow. The nurse on duty that night said she would monitor Aaron on a regular basis through the night, remembering he had a door in his room made me restless hoping he would not think to open it with the curtain closed disguising it.

At home I sat for a while surrounded by darkness not wanting to move, speak or in all truthfulness do anything. I could feel myself getting lower and lower in mood which scared me. The longer I sat the harder it got I didn't think I could feel so low but the last few months were finally taking hold of me. Nothing was going to defeat me, Aaron needed me, so until he was safe giving up was not an option.

Aiming to get back to Beechwood early the next morning anxious to see what sort of night Aaron had. Putting the last twenty four hours behind me I was ready for the challenge of the day. Driving into the car park I noticed his belongings were not at the front door, a good start Wednesday today hoping for some good news about Aaron's potential move.

Going to the nurse's station to get a run down on the nights events, all in all he slept most of it, not surprising the day he had he must have been shattered. Approaching his room where to my dismay there he was packing again, any elation I had just deflated making a suggestion to go into the therapy room to play a game or he could go into the dining room and make me a drink anything to stall for time. I was planning ways to distract him for as long as I could. The other two assessments were due to take place this morning. In my own mind I knew which unit would suit Aaron's needs, Oakleaf were keen to take him all that we were waiting for was the funding to be authorised. Once that had been approved it was all systems go. By mid morning Aaron was getting restless he started to walk towards the doors saying he was going out. As he approached them they didn't open, they had been locked which wasn't regular practice. The excuse was that they had a problem with them, but I knew it was to keep him in the last thing they wanted was a reoccurrence of yesterday. Not sure how long this could be kept up for before he twigged what was happening. Aaron then went to try the fire exit door, when challenged that he couldn't use that door he became aggressive and started to shout. What scared me most was that since his brain injury I was unaware of his capabilities in relation to the aggression and was not sure what form they would take.

A sense of relief came over me when I saw his family arrive they can now take over for a while, I can then focus on finding out what was happening. It was down to a phone call to decide Aaron's fate the call was to confirm if funding had been agreed.

But there was no news until Friday morning, I was literally on my knees how I have managed to get to today was beyond me. Since Wednesday we have all been trying to explain to Aaron that he will be moving but he needed to be patient, not something Aaron has to this day adapted well to.

It wasn't until lunch time on the Friday that Oakleaf called Beechwood with the news we'd all been praying for, everything had been approved. The only problem now was that Aaron could not be moved until Monday. Only two more day's the finishing post was in sight, giving Aaron the good news that he only had two more days left may calm him down. We were advised to visit Oakleaf before Aaron's arrival if we could to take a look around. The plan today was to go to Hartwell to do what was suggested. The drive to Oakleaf would take about half an hour as his parents arrived it was recommended that we take Aaron over there to get him away from the unit for a while. The drive was pleasant Aaron seemed to enjoy the drive, taking in all the sights. The gates to Oakleaf were closed when we pulled up and no one was answering the phone. The question was do we hang about or go back? Time was ticking so we headed back, I'll call them later to arrange a visit once Aaron was back at Beechwood, Which I did.

The photographs seen of Oakleaf Care on their web site did them no justice. Their location is on the outskirts of a village on top of a hill, it had a peaceful feeling. The gardens were a parade of colour uniform on their approach a great deal of care, love and pride had been put into them. The views were breathtaking over green fields that ran for miles. The poly tunnels were made up with rows of fruit and vegetables, pumpkins the size of beach balls sat idle in the corner. It was so quiet out here. There was nothing clinical about Oakleaf the staff were casual yet professional in their approach no uniforms were worn a sense of fitting in. The residents have the freedom to wander the internal grounds if an attempt is made to leave alarms will sound. Oakleaf Care was established in 2005, it offers high quality rehabilitation for adult males with acquired brain injury and associated physical and cognitive needs. All the staff are qualified and experienced in this area of care. They make sure all the residents are given all the opportunities open to them. For some of the residents this is their permanent home and they are all treated with dignity and respect. A better place I couldn't imagine and peace of mind that at least Aaron would be looked after and kept safe.

Monday could not come quick enough for me I hate having to wish my life away. The one thing we can never get back is time. But under the circumstances I think I deserve a little slack on that one.

The weekend was all planned trying to keep Aaron occupied until Monday. The days were packed with visitors taking shifts and the nights were left to the staff at Beechwood to make sure he was as safe as he could be. Trying to spend as much time with Aaron as I could but also trying to take time out. Saturday morning, the sun was shining the start of a very long weekend. On my arrival I was surprised to learn that Aaron had been helping one of the nurses in the dining room prepare for breakfast, he'd been courteous and smiling. Knowing he will be leaving in a couple of days seems to have cheered him up slightly. Keeping him occupied made him feel as though he was achieving something.

It filled me with sadness watching Aaron trying to complete tasks that before he could have done with no problems. Seeing the frustration and anger in his face as he did not understand why it's taking so long to do. Like trying to work out how the remote control works for the TV. The concept of time seems to be an issue as like a child when trying to appease them at Christmas time on how may sleeps there are left until the big day, seems to be the case with Aaron on how long before his move. I was looking forward not having to be on tender hooks all the time, my heart being in my mouth every minute. Another night of anxiety my stress levels must be ready to explode. The more I try to relax the more stressful I became.

Sunday followed much like Saturday Aaron was in a relatively good mood. Feeling relaxed today more than I have done since this nightmare began, cannot explain why, I know we both have a very long journey ahead, what that entails is yet to be seen I'm sure there are going to be plenty of ups and downs I just hope I can find the strength to do it.

Filled with trepidation on the forthcoming months, I hope and pray that the pieces of the puzzle will finally come together.

# Chapter Five

*Oakleaf Care*

*Preparing for home*

———❦———

1 0th August 2009 feels like only yesterday as I remember it very clearly. A day I thought would never arrive a week ago. As sense of relief all round today knowing that Aaron was being moved to a safer environment. He was due to leave for Oakleaf (Hilltop House) at lunchtime, knowing he was going I had a feeling he would be in a good mood.

Setting off early morning planning in my mind how the day would pan out. I was met at reception by Aaron a smile appeared on his face when he saw me, something I had missed seeing over the last few months. It warmed my heart and the issues of the last week were pushed to the back of my mind. Noticing clutched in his hands were some flowers, he looked so nervous as if on a first date. I suppose it must have felt strange to him he knew I was his wife but to what extent? After a little hesitation he gave them to me, but wanted them back straight away. It seemed as if he only wanted me to hold them for a while, like a child wanting their new toy back.

Staff commented on how polite he had been that morning a joy to be around, it was a shame it could not have been like that all the time. In a way it would be sad leaving, for me anyway I'd got to know the staff we had a good relationship and worked closely in giving Aaron the best care. Especially over the last few weeks when I began speaking to one or two relatives of other residents going through similar nightmares as me. Knowing I was not alone.

Aaron's bags had been packed first thing, no surprise there. It's a wonder they weren't packed last night and placed at the door ready. One last check around just to make sure there was nothing lurking before we set off. The time had now come to say our farewells Aaron could not have been out the doors quick enough, for me I wanted to thank everyone at Beechwood for their help and support over some very trying weeks and promised to return with Aaron once his recovery had progressed and he was on the right road.

This new adventure was exciting in a way, looking forward to Aaron having more to occupy his mind. Knowing now he would not be home in September in a way was good under the circumstances. He was on a twelve week trial then a review would take place. All being well and funding approved the issue now was how long will his recovery take? Pulling into the driveway at Oakleaf I don't know which one of us was more nervous. It was a pleasant day getting out the car I stood there a while noticing the peace and quiet. The front door to the house opened, we were greeted by staff and escorted inside. Aaron was shown to his room which was situated on the ground floor although he had climbed a flight of stairs he was not ready I felt yet to go it alone. His room was cosy with its own wet room which he seemed to like. We were given time to settle in and unpack before Aaron was shown around the grounds. He seemed keen so I hoped he'd participate in whatever was to be thrown at him. There were still some reservations on my part but over time they were laid to rest.

Everyone seemed really positive the resident's happy staff portraying a feeling of thoughtfulness. I was looking forward to see what they had planned for Aaron as far as rehab goes but I knew it would take a couple of weeks at least for that to be sorted. The problem was the more time Aaron had on his hands the worse he was, the last thing we needed was a repeat of the last week.

The afternoon was flying by as we sat in his room, just then a knock at the door. In walked Dan Gordon Deputy General Manager (now Rehabilitation & Liaison Manager), he introduced himself shook our hands and welcomed Aaron to Oakleaf. From that moment on I had a feeling Dan and I would get on well in the months to come, a sense that this was a man I could with any luck come to confide and trust in. It was his presence that struck me the most he spoke with great passion about Oakleaf and the role he played.

When Dan left I was left to fill out forms also a little time for us both to chill before dinner was served. Getting restless Aaron made his way to the lounge and sat down to watch TV, at that point one of the other residents's sat beside him. Looking at my watch I decided to leave to give Aaron time to get use to his new surroundings, be on his own for a while. Feeling sad as I left watching his face as I walked out, wondering what would happen if he followed me? Thinking how much longer before he'll be alright? After saying goodbye I just sat like a statue in the car tears uncontrollably just ran down my face, not sure why, was the fact of Aaron being away from home? The whole build up of the last week or was it the reality at that point was he ever coming home? Still didn't know much about brain injury each day was a new challenge but I became optimistic that I could learn more from Oakleaf.

Back home sorting things out back to work tomorrow first time for over a week. I was still on reduced hours but once Aaron was on a structured timetable visiting would be condensed, which meant I could not go until late afternoon. Good in one way I could concentrate more on work, myself and try and find my identity for that had seemed to be lost along the way. It was going to feel strange though, someone else caring for Aaron after it had been my role for a while. I think the hardest part of it would be to let go having a sense that he may not need me so much, but how can I get back the role of a wife when Aaron was at Oakleaf, was I to be in limbo? What do I do? I hadn't known that part of me for months.

After a couple of days everything seemed to be going ok, no unexpected dramas had unfolded yet but it's still early days. On a walk around the grounds we took some time to sit under the gazebo, looking over the miles of fields. Then walking through the stunning, colourful gardens, stopping to smell and admire their beauty. Aaron soon lost interest so back in we went he suggested going to the shop, when asked what he wanted he didn't seem to know. Trying not to be on his heels all the time the idea now he was at Oakleaf was to give him some freedom, knowing he was safe and couldn't just wander off. Sitting on the back itching to follow as he left the room, within seconds alarm sounded everywhere, quite deafening. Running out to find Aaron had got out of the front door, within seconds staff had congregated trying to coax him back inside. You could see he wasn't happy, swearing under his breath as he marched back to his room. He then started to take all the clothes out of his wardrobe and place them in his bag saying he was going home. Slowly attempting to talk him down the agitation came through. Thinking I can't go through this again. Knowing he could not leave eventually he calmed down. Was I to leave now or stay a bit longer? Wishing someone could tell me what to do? How much longer can this go on for? What if he's like this from now on? Panic set in and for a while I thought about getting in the car and not coming back, that's it no more. But how could I he didn't know what he was doing. How would I have felt if it was me in this position?

Each day that followed Aaron packed his belonging and tried to escape, when challenged by staff he would become agitated. What if this isn't the place for him? If after twelve weeks he's not suited at Oakleaf where then? I wanted to shake him and try and get through to him the importance of him being here. If that wasn't enough I was having challenges of my own at home, sorting out all of the finances now that we didn't have Aaron's wage coming in. It's a wonder I wasn't smoking fifty cigarettes a day along with a bottle of wine just to keep me going.

The weekend flew by before I left on Sunday Aaron decided to have a shave, standing in the bathroom watching him pick up his toothbrush trying to shave with it. Taking out the razor from his wash bag I put it in his hands explaining that's what he needs, but he was adamant he was right. It took a couple of minutes then he picked up the razor, you could see the concentration on his face, he knew what to do the motion of the shave on his face but somehow not working. It was then he attempted to put toothpaste on his face and shave that. Getting mad with me for interfering, what could I do just stand back? Teaching him was so hard when asked to pick up a comb he picked up the toothbrush again. I was to discover later that Aaron had Dyspraxia which I was told is common in brain injury. Dyspraxia is a learning difficulty that can affect the planning of movements as well as co-ordination as a result of brain messages not being accurately transmitted to the body. Dyspraxia is associated with memory problems especially short term memory therefore a sufferer can have difficulty remembering instructions. To them carrying out the simplest of tasks that require planning and sequencing can prove to be a big issue. But anyone who suffers with dyspraxia benefits from working in a structured environment by repeating the same routine on a regular basis, just as Aaron is doing.

It was sad seeing this but with time and practice surely this would improve?

A pattern was forming with Aaron he still made attempts to leave the house by setting off the alarms at any given chance he got, kept packing all his belongings until staff along with my consent decided to remove all his belongings out of his room taking temptation away from him. Then to make matters worse for Aaron he was placed under 24 hour observation. None too pleased at the prospect of someone following him around all the time made Aaron more agitated, he swore at staff at every opportunity then on the flip of coin was pleasant towards them. Whilst I visited he didn't need watching, he just turned his aggression towards me. He blamed me for leaving him there every day.

The walking stick that Aaron arrived with was soon taken from him surprised he didn't miss it. His walking got better every day he seemed to find this new confidence although it was still at a slow pace. All in all his physical being had greatly improved, if only his mind would catch up. I later discovered that Aaron was attending Taekwon-do sessions which astounded me Aaron has never been one to exercise. Maybe this is a new found skill that he may pursue.

Since his admission to Oakleaf Aaron had absconded a total of nine times. Due to this it was suggested that he be moved from the house into the lodge. It was felt that Aaron would suit the slower pace of life there. The lodge was smaller than the house, but still situated in the grounds of Hilltop but catered for residents who needed long term support. On the 10th September Aaron was moved. Here there was no view of the front door or the car park so not prompting him to leave as much. His new room was on the first floor, worried a little as stairs were involved but it didn't take long for him to get used to them. He was careful using the rails provided. The room itself was bright around the same size as the one in the house but the lodge was a newer build with a more comfortable feel. Aaron settled well and with all his belongings returned to him he did not attempt to leave again for a while. For me it was time to go back to work full time, Aaron had settled to a degree at Oakleaf. It was going to be good for me for me to get back some normality in my life may be the days would not feel so long.

It was fast approaching Aaron's first review at Oakleaf he still has no insight into his injury which makes him vulnerable and therefore how he behaves affects other if he was to be placed back into the community. I had concerns about it as not sure what happens, how and who is present but the main question was could they still help Aaron? To prepare me for the review I had a meeting with Dan pouring my heart out he responded with compassion and support as I thought he would. Reassuring me all would be ok all that was left for me to do was hang on for the review which was set for 22nd October 2009.

The day had finally arrived, review day strangely daunting being my first. Thirteen of us sat round a large table all of us deciding Aaron's future. Dan opened the meeting by explaining the procedure. Listening with interest to everyone in the room discussing how Aaron had been in the last three months, from the nursing to the Speech and Language side. It was noted how his move from the house to the lodge had been a surprising success. By now there was an idea of what Aaron required as far as rehabilitation goes, the only issue was getting him engaged. Aaron was still in the early stages of his assessments and rehab journey. It was felt that Oakleaf could offer Aaron support, structure and encouragement in the months to follow.

The review brought up areas of difficulty that Aaron was dealing with, Psychology being one of them. From their point of view and over a period of several sessions, most of which Aaron was not willing to engage in so many were taken from observations. His memory has been severely impaired due to his injury. He has poor concentration levels and problems understanding language due to his poor logical memory. Aaron tends to repeat or re-iterate that last thing he has seen or heard. It was also noted that significant Retrograde Amnesia (RA) was present. For example when asked how old he was he would responded 29, when in fact he was 39. RA is a loss of information of the past which in Aaron's case brought on by his injury. In severe cases a person can actually forget who they are. Thankfully as far as Aaron's concerned that hasn't occurred.

There was also an indication that Aaron had Ideomotor Apraxia (IMA), finding it difficult to mimic familiar tasks. One defining symptom of IMA is the inability to act using equipment. For example someone suffering from IMA was handed a comb they may try and move it around their head or even attempt to brush their teeth with it. Like with the motion of Aaron picking up his toothbrush to shave with.

In conclusion it is still early days as far as the Psychologist assessment goes therefore their aim was to encourage Aaron to take part in future sessions.

The meeting went on to discuss Occupational Therapy. Aaron's interests in this area to engage have been hindered by his insight to his injury. On his personal hygiene although independent there is still and area for improvement. There is no consistency to his pattern where personal hygiene is involved. Aaron was observed not using deodorant or cleaning his teeth on a regular basis, shaving when encouraged or by intervention by me.

Other actions where difficulties were observed were the making a hot drink a task he started to do at Beechwood. It was noted that Aaron had difficulty planning, preparing and sequencing the procedure. Many errors were evident of Apraxia. This is the loss of the ability to execute or carry out purposeful movement, despite having physical ability and the desire to perform such activities. With rehab there is no reason why Aaron should not improve.

On their conclusion it was evident that Aaron required a structured rehabilitation programme in a structured environment.

In relation to the Speech and Language Therapy (SALT) although Aaron had made some progress since coming to Oakleaf he is still very much disorientated and there may be a potential for him to decline rather than improve. Careful observation was needed this said it is severely affecting his ability in all area of his daily living, some of which have been mentioned. An area that was present which was to be considered was Post Traumatic Amnesia (PTA). This is a state of confusion that immediately follows a traumatic brain injury, where the sufferer is disorientated and unable to remember events that occurred after the injury. There are two types of amnesia one being RA, which has been previously touched on. Therefore it was advised as far as SALT is concerned ongoing rehab was essential for Aaron.

Half way through the meeting nothing I heard came as a surprise. Having been actively involved throughout Aaron's recovery I was pleased with all the reports so far. Up next was the assessment from the Physiotherapist who at this stage had not had a lot of dealings with Aaron due to his unwillingness to participate. Although Aaron has a full timetable, physical activity is very much encouraged. Unfortunately before his injury Aaron was not much into physical exercise so that didn't shock me. There were no major concerns as far as physiotherapy goes but Aaron will still be encouraged to take part to remain active.

One area I thought Aaron would find of interest was the Horticultural Therapy due to his interest in gardening back home. Having something familiar may encourage him to participate. Although he has attended sessions in this area he has needed a lot of encouragement but once attended he has completed the full session. He has gained a good rapport with staff, but I feel these sessions will be short lived on Aaron's part.

After the meeting a summary and recommendations were discussed. Over the next review period they were anticipating natural recovery to take place. Further assessments will be needed with continued monitoring to keep up with the changes Aaron will make. The next review had been set for three months time February 2010. It became apparent to me that although there were no surprises in the review, having listened to each area it was evident just how ill Aaron was. Using words such as Post Traumatic Amnesia or Apraxia meant nothing to me but sounded very scary. It hit home more having it down in black and white that his recovery according to these reports was going to take years, not months as I had naively thought. The plan was to research as much as I could on brain injury if I stood any chance of helping Aaron.

Every attempt was made by staff at Oakleaf to engage Aaron into sessions, with his timetable full there was nothing stopping him. However Aaron was stubborn it was not easy trying to encourage him into doing something he just didn't want to do. He felt there was no purpose to it especially with not having any insight into why he needed to do what was being asked of him.

Saturday 7th November Oakleaf have organised a firework display. I'm really looking forward to it. It's like the first outing as a couple since Aaron's injury the display would be taking place in the grounds of Oakleaf it was the thought of just getting out that appealed more. All wrapped up ready to go we made our way along with others to the end of the garden the bonfire was roaring in the field beyond the grounds. The smell of burgers being cooked, children running about, people talking felt normal. I held onto Aaron's arm just in case he decided to wander off. He seemed to be getting into the spirit although swearing under his breath at the passing children, trying not to let it ruin the evening we went for something to eat. Aaron is allergic to cheese but all he wanted to eat was a burger with cheese. When told he didn't like it that's when he changed, the agitation and frustration took over, shouting at me and anyone that spoke to him. The only thing to do was take him back inside. Staff came over and asked if all was ok, which made him worse. Trying to calm him down did not make him any better. As we walked back to the lodge not a word was spoken between us, glad in one way I think I would have exploded at him there and then. All it took was twenty minutes from going out to coming back in the shortest outing I've had. Not wanting to upset him any more I left feeling devastated. By now the light at the end of the tunnel was getting further away was it normal to feel this way? Hating myself for letting things get to me so much. Could not get home quick enough, once there I rang to see if he had settled. It seemed that he had forgotten all the events of earlier and was content just watching TV in his room. The rest of November came and went with no major changes as far as Aaron's rehab was going. It was still a constant battle trying to get him engaged all he wanted to do was hibernate in his room.

The month I'd been dreading has finally arrived, December everyone else around me seemed to be looking forward to the festive break for me I just wanted to crawl under a duvet and not come out until it was over. The nearer it got the more disheartened and depressed I became, not a tree or decoration was in sight at home. No one would be coming round so what was the point. Yes gifts were brought but I got no enjoyment from it. It was a chore to write out cards feeling a real bah humbug. I didn't even turn on the TV. I felt angry and jealous of others making plans and looking forward to the holidays. Having to pull myself together it could have been worse at least Aaron was here and we were spending the day together.

Christmas 2009 is one I will not hold with fond memories in the years to come. The week before the weather was bad, more snow than we have had before. Oakleaf had arranged a carol concert put on by the residents unfortunately due to the weather it had to be cancelled I had already booked the day off work to spend at Oakleaf. Good job really I would not have made it into work anyway. Looking out if the window I saw the car completely snowed in, great just what I didn't need. Putting me in a rotten mood before the day had begun. Knowing there was no way for me to get over to see Aaron the first thing that entered my mind was if I don't see him every day will he forget who I was? Knowing his memory was poor would he actually forget me? Not that it was likely but back then it is strange what goes through your mind. The thought of being trapped in the house alone for the whole weekend would drive me mad this was when I hit rock bottom. What made the situation worse was when I rang to try and speak to Aaron I was told by staff that his parents had arrived. Knowing they only live ten minutes from us got me thinking why had they not have called me to see if I could get there especially with the weather as it was. Literally breaking down on the phone my mind set on getting to Oakleaf. It was Staff on the other end that talked me down, glad they did there was no way I would have made the journey.

The day didn't get any better trying to occupy my mind made me feel even sorrier for myself than I already did. It got to the stage as night drew in sitting in the darkness thinking no more, I was so tired nothing else to give. The phone rang and rang didn't want to talk to anyone but I picked it up. Aaron's aunt was on the other end asking if I was ok, wrong thing to ask me. Half an hour later she was knocking on my door insisting she stay with me through the night. I cried that night until I could cry no more, I missed my dad and Aaron but not sure who the most.

The day had taken its toll on me so I was glad to see the back of it as dawn broke the next day. Waking up I was determined not to feel that low again. The only way I could describe the feeling was like being in a big, dark hole and each time I gripped on the sides to pull myself up the deeper the hole got. Not sure how I got out in the end but the strength came from somewhere. Honestly though if it hadn't been that time of year I probably would not have gotten so bad, who knows?

Well Christmas day's here from the second I woke to the moment I went to bed I have never wanted a day to go so quickly. At least with the house being Christmas free it felt like an ordinary day. Showered and dressed by 9 o'clock, car packed I was on my way. Everyone was happy when I got to Hilltop carols playing in the background residents sat around enjoying the atmosphere. Aaron as usual was in his room, he'd not even been down for breakfast yet. The plan was to get him up, showered, dressed and downstairs to join in today. Watching him open his presents with eagerness was a joy as he responded to each one. It was special for me as the week before staff had taken Aaron out shopping for presents, the gifts that he'd chosen for me were all his own doing. I suppose I have to count my blessings that Aaron was walking and talking, but watching him I could see this child like presence still taking over. I prayed that with time the man I married would come back.

We sat and ate dinner together a rare occurrence these days everyone was considerate, especially the staff they tried to make it as special as they could. After a few visitors earlier that morning the afternoon was all ours. At some point I knew I had to leave but not wanting to go home I was invited round friends for the evening. Being with friends was a nice and a welcome distraction watching the kids laughing with not a care in the world their only concern was what to play with next. With a full house I watched everyone play games and have a good time, trying to laugh on the outside but feeling so lonely inside.

At last Christmas and New Year are over next hurdle was Aaron's 40th birthday on 23rd January. The original plan before his injury was to go to Las Vegas a place that holds a fondness with him, maybe he will return one day. Aaron by now had let his appearance slip, not shaving, showering or bothering with his hair he was beginning to look old. No matter what was said to him he was adamant he was ok. The beard that had grown was grey his fingernails needed cutting it's like he had completely given up. He was slowly turning into a man I did not recognise and certainly not the man I married. With him looking and feeling this way it wasn't much of a birthday, friends and family gathered and ate cake. No input by Aaron at all I think whatever we did would not have worked that day.

Something needed to be done so a week later Dan and I took Aaron into town to get his hair and beard cut. A chance we took, not thinking he would go along with it but to everyone surprise no objections was raised. It was good to have Dan was there just in case Aaron made a scene. The going out in public was still very new to me and if anything did happen I don't think I would have coped. We sat waiting for Aaron's turn in the salon, he was calm observing what was going on with such interest. On first approach he looked perfectly normal whatever was going on inside his head. Sitting on the edge of our seats just waiting but all credit to him he behaved like a gentleman. Only swore twice but not in a threatening manner or towards anyone directly. The transformation was complete forgetting what he'd looked like as the long hair and beard had just taken over, I was beginning to see the old Aaron slowly emerge.

Aaron's next review was now approaching not so nervous this time. I had started to get to know the staff, we worked well together relaying information off each other so it was I felt more at ease this time round. The review was the same structure as the previous one so I knew what was coming.

11th February 2010 Aaron's second review, Dan was their chairing the meeting making sure each area was covered and explained. Since Aaron has been at Oakleaf he has had a named nurse assigned to him. His designated nurse had been changed since he moved over to the lodge. Although Aaron does not tend to engage with his named nurse it makes it difficult for them to get to know him. Since the last review although there have been improvements it is still evident that Aaron requires specialist rehabilitation. He still has problems attending his daily sessions, not through want of trying by staff that in turn makes the process of assessing Aaron more difficult. Due to his unwillingness to co-operate there is a rise in his confrontational behaviour, he is more likely to challenge staff when asked to perform a certain task or ask why? From there he will withdraw from the situation. However his personal hygiene has seen a vast improvement and a sign of awareness. The real challenge now is getting him to build relationships with the staff, he finds it difficult putting names to faces and he will only do this once trust has been gained. There is still a long way to go for Aaron with his rehab it was felt that Oakleaf was the best place for that journey. So it was decided to review him again in six months.

It's quite sad sitting round a table deciding the future of someone who is not there, not that Aaron would have been able to understand what was going on. It may take him time to gain the trust of the staff at Oakleaf but for me I've had to do that from day one. Making sure Aaron is being cared for and given the best opportunity that is on offer to him. Over time my trust in them has grown and I have come to value the work that they do.

Up till now since being in the lodge Aaron has not once mentioned about coming home, is it because he doesn't know where home is? Or simply because he knows that for the time being he cannot go home? It was devastating enough to know he could not remember our wedding day in 2004 or any events or our lives from then. I put together an album of photos with memorable dates in the hope that something might jog his memory. The trouble was no one could even tell me if any of the memories would return. All those years, gone all those memories erased for how long? I suppose it's time to try and build some new ones.

There was days in March and April coming up that for me hold significant memories, some of which are not so good, I could feel myself spiralling into depression again. It was getting to the stage where time out was needed for me to charge my batteries. For the last year all the time that I took off had been to do with Aaron. I somehow forgot how to just relax not to sound selfish, think of me. The anniversary of dad's death was looming in March also a year in April since Aaron's injury. On looking back the time has felt as if it's flown, yet not if that makes sense. Going through the motions each day my routine was getting predictable, work all day, then Hilltop. I was however finding more time to spend with friends, not on a regular basis but enough to get me started.

Another catch up with Dan was in order before I found myself back to where I was last December and believe me not a place to go. Dan carries a presence about him that makes him easy to talk to. Although Aaron was making slow progress his concerns were more for me. Since dad died and Aaron has been ill I find I have no male role to confide in, so Dan has been appointed that post becoming my rock and confidant, he gives me the strength to carry on.

Coming up I'd almost forgot my birthday which that year was on a Friday. Wanting to do something that included Aaron as I felt he had missed out on his birthday. The decision had been made to for the first time since his injury go out for a meal in a restaurant. Bit of a challenge but unless we tried how were we to know he could cope with it. It was all set then Aaron stated he wanted to spend the night at home. The only problem with that was if he did come home, would he go back? Speaking to Dan and staff at Oakleaf permission was required from the doctor. If he felt it was ok and Aaron was up to it then it would be all systems go. I got the call Friday morning from Dan to say he had just heard from the doctor to say Aaron had the all clear to come home. All that was required was his medication for the night a few things in a bag and all set. One condition was set for Aaron he had to return the next day. Filled with trepidation it too late to back out now, not sure how I was going to feel once he was home it's been over a year. How would he react?

On leaving Hilltop he promised to return however if a problem did arise Oakleaf would be there to support. So by lunch we were in the car on route for Rushden. Once home he paced about just looking around getting his bearings, going upstairs the cats looking at this stranger wandering about. He made his way into the kitchen it was there I asked him to make a drink, carefully observing his every move seeing how he would react to a totally different environment. Not knowing where to find anything he did ask, then once told it didn't take long for him to adapt. It felt strange having him there a sense that it was going to take time getting use to him in the house again. Half of me expected him to revert back to the old Aaron as soon as he walked in, when I knew that wasn't going to happen, the loss of how it used to be became unbearable. Hiding my emotions feeling just how raw this whole situation still is. It's funny but while he has been away I'm trying to cope the best way I can now that he's here I don't know what to do because deep down I know things will never be the same.

I was filled with anxiety going to the restaurant for the first time we went early to avoid crowds, hopefully by doing this it reduced the chances of Aaron becoming agitated. As this was one of Aaron's favourite places I knew he would enjoy it. The whole evening went surprising well no outbursts or frustration rose, when asked questions by the waiter he was polite and well-mannered. It was very pleasant although I could not completely relax knowing what I knew about him.

Once the meal was over I didn't want to hang about glad to get in the car and head for home. It was really bizarre having him there he had become a stranger. Perceiving how tired Aaron got it wasn't long before he wanted to go to bed, his medication given so all that was left was to get through the night. I was conscious he was in the house it wasn't long before thoughts turned to wonder what will happen if he had a fit? The staff at Oakleaf had run through the procedure if one occurred but was I really prepared? Each time he moved or woke up I was like a cat on a hot tin roof, watching every hour on the clock pass by. Is this what it would be like if he came home? I was exhausted and it was only one night. Taking into account how confusing it must have been for Aaron, all he had known was Hilltop. Morning had arrived he wanted to go and get his hair cut, usually he went on his own so when I tagged along he looked at me wondering why I was going with him. Walking into the barbers he had to wait a while. Working as quick as they could it wasn't long before it was his turn. Was I to mention to them the problem with Aaron or say nothing? When they asked him what he wanted he couldn't explain. I then stood up went and stood behind him and explained for him, sat back down, my heart was beating so fast I'm sure the chap next to me could hear it. It was then that Aaron looked at me and said "what do you know" loud enough for all to hear. Just wanting the floor to open and swallow me up, all I could do was look away, thinking don't get upset, not here, not now then getting mad with him in my mind thinking "how dare you speak to me like that after all I've done" wanting to shout it at the top of my voice.

It was going to be a long day he was expected back at Hilltop just after lunch, thinking it would be a relief once he's back, does that sound horrible of me thinking that? There was no way I could have him home full time not yet

I wasn't physically or emotionally prepared for it. As much as I loved him it would not work not the way he was.

Once the football had finished on TV he said "let's get back" this had been a lot harder than I thought it would be and made me realise just how much of an impact his brain injury has had on our lives. Arriving at Hilltop staff asked if all was ok, Aaron would not speak to any of them but I stopped and spoke which angered him, "why are you telling them everything" was his response they were keen to know the outcome for future reference. Not staying long I said my goodbyes and left.

Travelling back alone in the car felt really strange back to an empty house again it felt like the last 24 hours didn't happen.

Now that he got a taste for home there was no stopping him he wanted to come home every weekend. Who can blame him surely being at home would be good for his recovery being surrounded by familiar things aiding his rehab. So who was I to say no this is what we were working towards. It was all well and good this happening but would it get to a point when he would refuse to go back? Was it a risk worth taking? From a selfish point of view I was in two minds about this, yes it would be good having him back home but as he was it wasn't going to be easy. The time I had at weekends to myself before visiting would stop so other sacrifices would have to be made. Being alone 24 hours a day for the whole weekend was a different ball game. All I could do was try so it was all arranged weekends home became a regular occurrence. Much harder than I imagined there would be times when I would forget Aaron's restrictions on what he was capable of, expecting him to do what he did before. At first I was watching his every move, when he walked out of a room I would follow, becoming obsessed. By the time he went back on a Sunday afternoon I was totally shattered then up for work the next day it got to the point where I didn't know if I was coming or going. My visits in the week to Hilltop had to be reduced I physically could not keep up.

Its funny how you start to forget how life used to be, dwelling on the past trying to recreate it doesn't work. Over time people change anyway it's making the best of what you have. As far as Aaron was concerned he was alive and getting better each day. Other residents at Oakleaf were not as fortunate as Aaron. Counting my blessings it was time to rebuild a new life.

Having Aaron home at weekends during the summer months seemed to do him the world of good, keeping him as occupied as much I could, knowing that when he returned to Hilltop his stubbornness would re appear and engaging him in his sessions would reduce. Getting the idea I could get him interested in the garden at home may make him enthusiastic and want to continue this in the week. He probably thought the weekends at home would be a doddle and I would just run around after him, wrong. I imagined sometimes he went back on a Sunday for a rest. There were days though when his agitation and frustration surfaced I was the only one there for him to take it out on. Not wanting to shout back or challenge him I hid away sobbing, locked in the bathroom or bedroom. Many times I could have easily left without looking back thinking let someone else deal with it. Living with someone that has a brain injury is so different from just visiting them for a couple of hours. I really don't think anyone can get a true reflection of just how hard it is for the carer, particularly a husband or wife.

Couple of months have now passed and Aaron's third review was due, getting used to them now. The review this time was chaired by Kathy Swannel, Clinical Director at Oakleaf, Aaron's named nurse and staff from their field of expertise. It's 5th August 2010 with the review underway it was reported that Aaron's communication has seen an improvement. However he does tend to become angry and agitated when his speech deteriorates, therefore it was felt that his speech and language therapy was of a priority.

Although Aaron had made some improvements staff had noticed a heightened level of verbal aggression, which I'm told is expected when he becomes more aware of his situation and insight increased. With this in mind my main concern was how Aaron would cope once the realisation of what has happened to him takes hold, would all the hard work that has been done be forgotten. Would his heightened agitation take on a different form? With a lot of uncertainty ahead I had a feeling it would be a rocky road in the months ahead.

As far as Occupational Therapy goes they have seen an improvement in Aaron. He has finally accepted one of the therapists who have worked really hard to gain his trust. He is beginning to open up to some of the therapy that they offer. It was however stressed in the report that when Aaron is out in the community it is vital he is never alone, being vulnerable due to his injury could potentially cause problems if he becomes irritated or aggravated.

During the review I commented that since Aaron has been coming home at weekends there has been much that I have learnt through advice from staff. One change that has occurred with Aaron is that he has begun to handle money, getting to understand the concept again. When out shopping getting him to go and purchase goods on his own, hand over money seeing him give the right amount. Also going to the bank to use the ATM is going ok although he does sometime get the numbers mixed up. At home he has begun to use the computer checking e-mails. At the beginning he would ask how to open them, delete them and close the computer down. After a couple of weeks he shouted at me for watching him claiming he was capable of doing it himself. I think he just wanted to feel independent and in control of something.

There seemed to be a general feeling of unity within the room, everyone was beginning to understand just where Aaron was and looking to increase the level of rehab by challenging him more. Psychology report next the therapists carrying out assessments on Aaron were having problems getting him out of his room to do the sessions. He occasionally would come across sarcastic but had a good sense of humour in general. There was a sense that Aaron felt safe when in his own surroundings. Aaron was not always consistent when it came to his rehab he was still a proud man and if he felt as though he was failing in something he just sooner not do it. On visits I would ask what he had done that day, most of the time he'd say nothing. Trying to convince him he needs to do his session he'd reply "why, they don't do me any good" he knew he could shower, dress and make hot drinks why did he have to prove he could do them. This is when it became difficult explaining to him why he was there when he felt he didn't. Acceptance of knowing exactly what had happened to him had not made sense to him yet. It was funny if we were out in the community and someone that he knew approached him and asked how he was, if it was someone he had not seen in a while he would say he had been in hospital with a bad arm, leg or back. Not once did he say I've had a brain or head injury. Was it because he generally did not know or was it because he did not want to accept what had happened to him?

Back to the review even though there had been some progress made further goals needed to be met, practically behavioural issues. Aaron needs time still to build relationships with staff, which at the moment is affecting his co-operation but all encouragement will be made to try to keep him focused and engaged. So another 6 months at Oakleaf for Aaron which was welcomed by me, just hoping Aaron can see it's in his best interest. By then it will be February 2011 coming up for nearly 2 years since his injury. Early days as far as brain injuries go but a life time for those affected.

I started to restrict my visits to Hilltop Aaron was doing well if there were any problems I knew staff at Oakleaf would call me. With him coming home at weekends it gave me an opportunity to have some time for me now. It became apparent with Aaron that he was starting to mention coming home more and seemed convinced that when he had got his eye sorted out he would be home. Since his injury there has been a problem with Aaron's left eye, hospital visits were ongoing to try and get this rectified.

He honestly believed that's why he was at Oakleaf. It was mentioned on numerous occasions to him that his eye was not the problem but he was certain it was. We had talked about him having a longer period at home this Christmas but concerns were now at the forefront of everyone's mind that he would not come back this time. A meeting was arranged between me, Dan and the doctor to speak openly to Aaron to try and get through to his stubborn side exactly why he was there and what was expected of him before being allowed home. Thinking the chat had got through to him it was all set for him to come home for eleven days over the Christmas period a real test for all. Looking back over the last year seeing how far he had come knowing this year would not be a repeat of the last one. A chance to look forward, the house for a while will become a home again, filled with noise and life.

Hoping I would survive eleven days I began to get ready for Christmas, a challenge was to see if Aaron could go into the loft to get all the decorations down, I don't do lofts, if it was left to me there would have been nothing. Watching as he prepared the ladder and climb up, making sure each footstep was carefully taken trying not become too fanatical. It came as second nature for him he could not see the fuss being made when he was finally down. The more Aaron had to think about a task the harder it became to carry it out. Noticing how he dealt with going up into the loft shows the rehab is working. Along with Aaron being at home my mum was also due to visit, this would prove interesting as she had not seen Aaron in a while so it would be fascinating to find out just how much he has progressed from her point of view.

Bringing him home for Christmas his bag was packed making sure he had what he needed he made the comment of "well if I haven't got it I will see it when I come back", relief knowing he was coming back. Armed with his medication for the duration we were off. There was something exciting about this break and it would give me true indication on how he we both would cope for a longer period.

Even though we had plans over the Christmas period the majority of time was spent alone, I felt more relaxed and tried to give him more freedom around the house, this time mainly for my own sanity. Being able to leave him on his own for short periods of time was becoming more frequent, something that I've found difficult to do in the past. There were a couple of incidents where Aaron became agitated when questioned about these he did not remember. Being too hard on myself feeling guilty to a degree by not praising him enough for all the progress he had made concentrating far too much on the negatives and not on the positives. All in all the break was a success but it has left me ready for another one.

New Year and determination set in that this one was full of optimism. Nothing can get as bad as the previous years and for once I wasn't going to let it. Aaron was slowly on the mend more challenges lie ahead feeling stronger, not afraid to challenge Aaron when he is in the wrong the year began well.

Over the first few weeks back at Hilltop Aaron's mood started to change, he became withdrawn and depressed. January deemed by some as not one of the best months, dark nights, cold weather, not much to look forward to so after his long stint at home was there any wonder he was struggling to get back into a structured routine. Staff felt as though they were going back finding it hard to get Aaron motivated and engaged. Sharing my concerns with Dan he decided to sit Aaron down talk to him to find out just where he saw himself heading. Aaron can be very strong minded as well as confrontational at times Dan discovered that his main aim was to come home. It was a compromise between them on how to move forward. Aaron was told what was expected from him whilst at Oakleaf. There seemed from that point a transformation overnight Aaron began to attend sessions, becoming more polite to staff it was a pleasure watching the old Aaron finally start to emerge.

Towards the end of January I met up with Dan he suggested Aaron be moved into community housing he felt it was the next step for him to built his independency and gain more control by having to fend for himself more. Once the proposal had been mentioned to management at Oakleaf and approved, plans would then be put into place for the transfer to begin. They knew just where to re house Aaron a new community residence had just been built. The location was nearer to home and would provide Aaron with the recovery he needed. It was agreed not to disclose to Aaron for the time being as we were not sure how he would react. Further discussions would take place on his next review set for 2nd February 2011.

Convinced it was a good move I felt very optimistic going into the review, discussing how further improvements had been made there was still a long way to go. Reading the report it indicated that Aaron does not show any pleasure interacting with other, especially where he resides. Hoping his move to community housing will rectify this, being with residents that will be as independent as him. The location will be a more relaxed, homely environment with only four other males living there hoping Aaron will open up more.

The review process is an opportunity to assess the progress of not just Aaron but all residents, making sure everyone is given the best possible chance to have a quality of life that most of us take for granted. A team of experts work together in their specialist area to share their knowledge and aim to move forward with those suffering from brain injury. I have been privileged to have been able to work with these people, amazed by their enthusiasm and drive to succeed in the recovery of such a horrific disability. It's good being involved with the staff at Oakleaf knowing we are all coming from the same mind set where Aaron's rehabilitation is concerned. Even though the reports show a remarkable recovery it is extraordinary due to the fact that his rehab programme has not been consistent due to Aaron lack of participation. The main recommendations are to keep the rehabilitation going making sure Aaron achieves his ultimate goal of going home, however I feel that as insight into his injury takes hold of him there are more obstacles ahead.

Along with all this Aaron has been having regular visits to hospital in relation to his left eye. Unable to see out of it since his injury we have now been informed that the only option for him is surgery.

It's like we have come full circle when I first heard that Aaron had to go back to John Radcliffe to have his eye operated on a sense of trepidation fell over me. How uncanny going back to where it all started, this time though when it comes to leaving I will be bringing him home. The reason for Aaron having to have surgery is that when the bleed occurred in his head some of the blood went down behind the back of his eye and congealed there, causing him to have limited sight. At the time we thought he had double vision due to the brain injury. He was then told by an optician that he had cataract and until it could be rectified Aaron was given glasses that he never wore as he claimed they made no difference. In some cases the blood disperses, in others the only option is surgery. On a number of visits to Northampton Hospital we were told that the best surgeon to carry out the operation was based at Oxford. Without sounding strange I wanted to go back, how I was feeling then would be completely different to how I am now. I suppose I'm in a much better place emotionally, physically and mentally. Wanting to know if Aaron could remember anything about Oxford, not that it bothered me it was mainly to satisfy my own curiosity. However I did have a few reservations about the operation thinking of what have gone on previous. But I'm sure if there were any doubts I'm sure it would have been brought up before now.

On the day of the operation I woke with a feeling of butterflies in my stomach, slightly anxious but positive for Aaron mainly as this is what he has been waiting for. He didn't have to be at Oxford till 1130hrs so at least the traffic would be lighter. The downside is that we would hit it on the way back. Picking him up I asked if he was nervous, he replied "not at the moment but I will when I get there" perfectly understandable. A member of staff from Oakleaf followed behind just in case I needed assistance after the operation, like getting Aaron into the car as I was unsure how he was going to react to the anaesthetic, plus I needed a little support. Pulling into the hospital it felt as though time had stopped and that it had not been nearly two years since I was last here. Once parked and after checking in Aaron was shown to a bed on the ward and told that he would be seen shortly, this was the start of a very long day. All credit to Aaron he remained tolerant and in good spirits throughout the whole ordeal. Watching the coming and goings kept us entertained for a while, Aaron prepared himself in the fetching hospital gown. After needing a degree to adjust the bed, he was settled once more, all we had to do now was hang around waiting for Aaron to have his blood pressure and temperature taken. By mid afternoon an orderly appeared pushing a wheelchair he came to collect Aaron I could feel my heart beating faster, I felt sick to my stomach, this is it. I was having a conversation in my head convincing myself that he would be ok he was in good hands, what could go wrong? They do this every day, trying to stay optimistic my role for a while was now done for a while. An hour and half later we went back up to the ward looking round the curtain to see if he was back, the bed was empty. The nurse claimed he was in recovery and was ok. Sitting patiently he appeared with a smile on his face, eye patch over his left eye, hair sticking up looking like he'd put his fingers in the electric socket. The relief was indescribable he'd got through it that's all that mattered.

I asked if he was ok, he certainly looked it, whatever they had given in it's a pity they cannot bottle it, no sickness on his part which was good. The nurse asked Aaron if he would like a cup of tea and something to eat, an expression of eagerness took over his face, he must have been ravenous. He started to shake I touched his arm he felt cold, I pulled the blanket over him and knew as soon as he had drunk and eaten he would start to feel better. I was just grateful he was back in one piece so to speak. He tucked into the chicken sandwich and drank the piping hot tea hoping he wouldn't have to hang about too long. Looking over at the nurse's station they were sorting out his prescription, we were also waiting to speak to the surgeon to find out if the procedure went according to plan, but was told he would be in theatre for some time. I'm sure if the operation had not gone well someone would have notified us. Aaron was discharged once he was given the all clear by the nurse. An appointment had been arranged for us to go back to Northampton Hospital the following day for a check up. Armed with eye drops and pain killers we set off for home. Looking at my watch it had been just over seven and a half hours since we arrived. I was shattered. The journey as predicated took longer so by the time we hit Rushden it was nearly eight o'clock. Aaron on the other hand was full of life, knowing we had to be up early the next morning I went off to bed and left Aaron downstairs. Feeling more relaxed at leaving Aaron on his own a few months ago I would have stayed up until he was ready to go to bed. It just shows how within less than a year the progress and development he has achieved. I suppose because I see him nearly every day I don't notice it as much so when someone who has not seen him in a while give constructive feedback makes it all worthwhile. His eye will take a while to heal and regular follow ups to the hospital will hopefully prevent any additional problems in time I pray he regains full eye sight.

It's been an extraordinary journey one I don't believe for one moment is over, would I do it all again knowing what I know? Probably I would.

Brain injury does not affect everyone the same, each individual has a different recovery rate and their outcome may not be the same as the next sufferer. Some to a degree can make a full recovery whilst others may never be the same again. Even writing this book there is probably no one that has gone through exactly what Aaron or I have. But the one thing we all have in common is that we share our lives with brain injury, it becomes part of us whether you are a sufferer or a loved one. Lives have to be adapted with considerable changes that sometimes family cannot cope with. For them a choice has to be made, no one can tell you how to choose but whatever the decision you will know it was for the right reasons.

# Afterword

So what happens next? I wish I knew If only I could wave a magic wand to predict the years ahead. I don't know myself what the future holds but whatever is decided I want to look back and say "I did my best" without any regrets. Throughout all of this I know that there was nothing else I could have done to change what happened. All I did was to try and make the best of a terrible situation. Life can be cruel at times but we have to look at the things we have instead of what we don't have. It's easy to moan about trivial things and yes we have all been guilty of it at times, but when you really look at life and the things you achieve and gain that's what you take with you, not material possessions. If anything this last four years have taught me that life is precious and we must cherish it, we are not here for long and the people we meet along the way who touch our hearts and the paths we take mould us into who we are and what we do.

I wouldn't say that life is "back to normal" although I don't worry as much as I did. Wrapping Aaron in cotton wool has now subsided, but having him home every weekend is hard work and tiring, but less demanding than they were in the beginning. The good thing is now I can leave him for short periods of time on his own in the house. Going out is still hard as I'm not quite comfortable with him being alone. People only see the exterior of Aaron and physically you would not think there was anything wrong, which at times can be a disadvantage. Brain injury is known as the "hidden disability" so unless you are in a wheelchair or have some physical weakness members of the public will assume all is ok. So when Aaron becomes agitated and frustrated when out it can cause problems and can be quite difficult to control. Walking on egg shells is a constant feeling, not so much now but when Aaron first came home at weekends I had to think of where we could go. How busy would it get? What time should we go? How long for? Luckily after nearly a year of him coming home and the more Aaron goes out in the community the better he becomes.

Some say it's the loved ones that are the real victims of brain injury as there is likely to be more insight into the injury than the sufferer itself. No one can prepare you for a brain injury and no one can tell you how to deal with it.

I still have constant battles with myself over what I feel and to this day I still don't know what to do. There are still times even at the weekends when Aaron is at home that I take myself off into another room and just cry, my head buried in a pillow or towel thinking to myself I cannot do this anymore, feeling trapped is this what it's going to be like from now on? Maybe somewhere buried instinct will let me know what to do. Although I have come this far things change, people change and over the last two years both of us have changed in a way. Even though Aaron still tries to battle with his mind I cannot help but wonder what would of happened if I did not stay?. My feelings over the months have changed and although I still love Aaron it's a different kind of love. After feeling pain, anger, hurt, guilt and resentment to joy, relief and elation anyone who has been in this position would also have problems dealing with what they feel. I cannot blame anyone for giving up. I cannot judge anyone, no one can pass judgement until you have experienced a situation like this or similar. Nobody knows what really goes on. I have given the last two years everything, but sometimes when you get nothing in return it makes life hard and lonely. Aaron still finds it hard to show emotion but I am hoping in time it will return. To be honest I may be too frightened to leave now in a way. Part of me wants to stay but there is still a part of me that wants to go. It scares me in case I do not get all the feelings back for Aaron that I once had. I suppose we both have to learn to get to know each other all over again. I haven't yet spoken to Aaron to find out how he feels, the time just does not seem right, also not sure he would fully understand at this point on how he does feel. I know that he loves me, but has his love changed? I have had great support from friends throughout this. I speak to my mum every day without fail, no matter what sort of day I have had. Then there has been the great support from Oakleaf Care, especially Dan who has been my rock and whom I have depended on maybe too much at times. Have you ever thought that when you meet someone for the first time you get a gut feeling about them, that you know you are going to get on? That's what I felt the first time I met Dan back in August 2009. Whether that's just a sixth sense a women gets or not, but so far it's not let me down yet. Also during this whole life changing incident it was probably meant to be that I meet lifelong friends along the way.

It's been two years now Aaron continues to heal and I am still by his side thankful for each day that he is here. It looks as though we still have a long battle ahead, but some days get easier to bear. I'm not sure how long it's going to take Aaron to recover, if he ever will from his brain injury. I know life will never be as it was so no use trying to look back. With help and support from family, friends and Oakleaf Care Aaron continues to improve each day. I don't know what the future holds all I can do is look at the here and now, focus on each day.

Someone asked me why I called the book lost, well three reasons. Firstly because Aaron has lost part of his life, so doing the book was an opportunity for him to understand just what he and I had been through. Secondly for the last two years I have felt really lost at times, the fear was I did not know what was going to happen and not sure what I was going to do and still don't. Thirdly whilst Aaron was in the coma for three weeks we had the radio on and each day Michael Buble's "Lost" would play, listening to this it soon became apparent the words became significant to me.

With my life solely surrounded by brain injury this last two years I feel now it's time to give something back. Voluntary work is something I have been considering, giving a little time to people less fortunate, just to sit with them and make their day seem brighter is priceless.

So now that this chapter of my life is about to end and a new one begins I would like to sit back contented with life and not feel lost anymore. When that will be is yet to be known. All of the feelings from devastation to elation in the last few years have been at times more than I could bear.

So to finish I'd like to say in the words of Vinnie Jones:

"It's been emotional"

# Acknowledgments

There are so many people I would like to thank at this stage that have helped and supported me through this very difficult time, emotionally, physically and mentally. This experience has helped me come to terms with our life now. I also feel what has happened has made me a stronger person and I feel I can cope with anything that is thrown in my direction. All the people mentioned below deserve a special appreciation from me for helping to put Aaron back together with their dedication and support because without them he would not be here today.

Firstly I want to thank Tanya Denman, my neighbour for without her on the day of Aaron's injury I don't think I would have coped with the situation whilst waiting for the paramedics. Who when arrived took over and worked fast to get Aaron to hospital.

Next I'd like to thank all the A&E staff at Kettering General Hospital whose quick thinking saved Aaron's life. Also to the staff in the High Dependency Unit whom I got to know quite well when Aaron was transferred back there in June

2009. I spent the majority of my time caring for Aaron, feeding and changing him with their help also trying to be a wife by just sitting at his bedside.

All the staff at John Radcliffe Hospital in the NICU department & Neuro ward from all staff, Physiotherapists, Occupational Therapist and the full medical team who were Aaron's guardian angels for 3 weeks when he was in a coma fighting for his life, not just with the brain injury but pneumonia as well. Truly dedicated staff and saying thank you just does not seem enough.

A special thanks to all my friends and colleagues at Bedfordshire Police who kept me focused on my work, which at times was a welcomed distraction. The force has supported me especially the department that I work for throughout this difficult time. I have worked for Bedfordshire Police for over 11 years and I have to say it has been one of the best organisations I have worked for.

Beechwood Rehabilitation Unit is the next thank you on my list, all the staff from nurses to kitchen staff were there for me all hours of the day and night as Aaron's rehabilitation began. It was here that Aaron began to walk again and for that I am grateful. Whilst there Aaron's cognitive state was difficult he did not know where he was and why. The staff were on hand to support and help not just Aaron but me as well.

Oakleaf Care—Specialist Brain Injury Rehabilitation Unit (Hilltop House & Weston Favell) The staff's dedication and professionalism are outstanding and it has been an honour working with the team. They hold a special place in my heart and they have become my second family, Hilltop House & Weston Favell my second home. Oakleaf Care has been Aaron's place of residence since 10th August 2009. But it's Dan Gordon (Rehabilitation & Liaison Manager) I especially want to thank for without him to keep my feet on the ground I would have given in and walked away before now. With his integrity and compassion he has become important to me whilst Aaron has been there. He holds a wonderful gift within and should be proud of what he does. I have grown a deep respect and admiration for Dan and I am blessed to know him. He has kept me sane throughout this difficult time. His knowledge and experience on brain injury is vast and when I thought there was no hope, he would sit me down, talk to me and give me the strength and inspiration to carry on, so to you Dan a special thank you.

Everyone at Oakleaf Care is still continuing to help Aaron with his rehabilitation, how long for is unknown but I know he is in the best place to make that recovery.

Aaron's family—Val, Dave, Glynis, Richard & Sarah.

Andrew & Michelle Ellis—Who from day one have been there for both of us. They kept me fed and watered in the first 3 weeks each night when I returned from the hospital, their three girls, Alicia, 8 Naomi, 6 and Hannah, 4 were a wonderful sight. Their innocence and carefree attitude put a smile on my face and I wished when I was with them that I could go back to being that age so I could believe in nothing bad, just princesses.

Aaron's friend Matthew Woods (Woody)

To all my friends you know who you are, when I would be sat at home in the dark you would know when to ring and try and cheer me up.

Last of all to my mum, Richard my brother, sister in law Sue and the kids, I love you, this has been hard for us all especially after losing dad, but we are getting there.

# References:

Headway

Helpline telephone number: 0808 800 2244

Their mission is to promote understanding of all aspects of brain injury and to provide information, support and services to people with a brain injury, their families and carers.

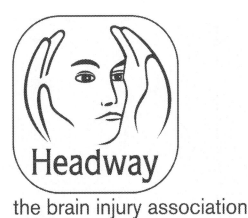

the brain injury association

www.headway.org.uk

Brain & Spine Foundation

Helpline telephone number: 0808 808 1000

www.brainandspine.org.uk

Stroke Association

Helpline telephone number: 0303 3033 100

www.stroke.org.uk

NHS

www.nhs.uk